# Intermittent Fasting for Women Over 50

The Simplified Guide to Lose Weight in A Simple Way, Promote Longevity, Increase Energy & Support Hormones with A Gentler Approach.

*by*

## Clara Grant

# Disclaimer Notice

Please note the information contained in this document is for educational and entertainment purposes only. All effort has been executed to present accurate, up to date, and reliable, complete information. No warranties of any kind are declared or implied. Readers acknowledge that the author is not engaging in the rendering of legal, financial, medical, or professional advice. The content in this book has been derived from various sources. Please consult a licensed professional before attempting any techniques outlined in this book.

By reading this document, the reader agrees that under no circumstances is the author responsible for any losses, direct or indirect, which are incurred as a result of the use of the information contained in this document, including, but not limited to, — errors, omissions, or inaccuracies.

or monetary loss due to the information contained in this book. Either directly or indirectly. You are responsible for your own choices, actions, and results.

# Table of Contents


**Introduction**

**Understanding Intermittent Fasting**

What is the Intermittent Fasting Diet? 11

History of Intermittent Fasting Diet 12

Why for ladies Over 50? 14

Why Should Women Choose the Intermittent Fasting Diet?

15

**Types of Intermittent Fasting**

16:8 Intermittent Fasting Method 17

5:2 Intermittent Fasting Method 18

Alternate Day Fasting (ADF) Method 20

Eat Stop Eat Intermittent Fasting Method 21

The Warrior Diet 23

One Meal each day (OMAD) Diet 24

**The Benefits of Fasting for Women Over 50**

Activating Cellular Repair 26

Increase Cognitive Function and Protects the Brain from Damage 27

Weight Loss   27

Alleviates Oxidative Stress and Inflammation   28

Slow Down the Aging Process   28

**Balancing Hormones and Increasing Energy**

Hormones   31

Energy   35

**Getting Started**

Fasting Plan for 5:2 Combined With 12:12   40

Non-Fasting Days   42

**7-Day Intermittent Food Plan**

Day 1 — Fasting Day 500 Calorie Allowance   46

Day 2 — Non-Fasting Day 2 000 Calorie Allowance   47

Day 3 — Non-Fasting Day 2 000 Calorie Allowance   48

Day 4 — Fasting Day 500 Calorie Allowance   50

Day 5 — Non-Fasting Day 2 000 Calorie Allowance   51

Day 6 — Non-Fasting Day 2 000 Calorie Allowance   53

Day 7 — Non-Fasting Day 2 000 Calorie Allowance   54

**Ideas for Healthy Eating**

Eating Nutritiously for ladies Aged 50 and Over   57

Healthy Eating Ideas 68

Healthy Breakfast Ideas 71

Healthy Lunch Ideas 78

Healthy Dinner Ideas 86

Healthy Smoothies 95

Beverages In Fasting Periods 105

Concerns In Fasting 108

## Dealing with Unpleasant Side Effects

Hunger 116

Frequent Urination 118

Headaches 118

Cravings 119

Heartburn, Bloating, and Constipation 120

Binging 121

Low Energy 122

Feeling Cold 123

Mood Swing 124

Bottom Line 124

## Changing Your Habits and Achieving Your Goals

Take Control of Your Habits                126

Breaking Bad Habits                         127

Switching the Bad for the Good              129

Change Your Mindset                         130

Have a Transparent Vision                   131

Chart Your Progress                         133

Set Obtainable Goals                        133

A New Daily Routine                         134

Create a Replacement Schedule               137

It Is All Up to You                         139

**Conclusion**

# Introduction

Expectations are a strong force! As people get older, they almost welcome physical and mental deterioration.

To some extent, wear and tear do happen to our bodies with time because we are using it at full capacity every day. But much of the decline in stamina may be a direct result of our minds. Society perceives older adults as weak, fragile, and "on their answer." Seniors themselves come to simply accept these perceptions and expect their bodies to start out showing signs of decline like bone density loss, lower muscle mass, high or low vital signs, slower metabolism, accumulated body fat, problems with blood glucose tolerance, achy joints, and so on. The strength of the mind can wield tons of power over the body!

These self-limiting beliefs make people take measures that will be detrimental to their health or ignore it, thinking it'll improve on its own. Suppose you feel that you grow older. Then it's inevitable to lose muscle mass, accumulate fat around the waist, and also discover more wrinkles, spots on the skin, and other flaws linked to getting old. So you're unlikely to interact in healthy habits to repair them. But once an individual can change their perception of aging, they're going to have the motivation to take deliberate keeping their body in sound health for the remainder of their life. One such action is fasting.

It is common for ladies approaching their golden age to harbor a secret fear of losing the vitality and wonder of youth. Some women want to avoid this point, just like the plague, due to concerns about not having the ability to remain healthy, sexy, and attractive. But all that fear makes no sense because it's possible to retain strength, intelligence, soft and tender skin, vibrancy, and every one the essential qualities of a healthy woman as long as she engages in the right habits. By implementing these suggestions and proposals, you'll begin to fall crazy with this particular time in life.

Coming aged isn't synonymous with inability, and this book will prove that to you! But beyond superficial proof, you'll be learning new healthy eating habits to make you look and feel younger than your biological age. Weight loss could seem just like the only proclaimed advantage of intermittent fasting, but you'll discover that there are advantages to a correct diet that transcend weight loss.

Your overall health and wellbeing aren't just suffering from what you eat, but once you eat. Immediately you would possibly be thinking it's pointless to start a replacement eating habit as an older adult. These thoughts are what put your health in a perpetual state of decline, plus it's never too late, especially for something which will improve your quality of life.

Intermittent fasting is quickly becoming the "it" thing for people of various age ranges. Many, especially young adults, are frothing over the thought of a replacement, quick, cost-effective thanks to reducing and are wanting to try it for themselves. This mentality is driven by the necessity to remain current or remain "on brand" with their social media presence. The downside is that folks get on a trend without doing their homework to retain the right knowledge and risk. This book overrides the fad mentality and can present you with unbiased information about intermittent fasting, mainly because it relates to women over 50. I even have removed unnecessary information irrelevant to those outside this age range so that older adults can have something to relate to.

Getting older may be a wonderful experience every woman should anticipate and celebrated as not everyone has the choice. It's my sincere hope that after reading these pages, you'll find the motivation to use what you've got learned and reap the various benefits of controlling your diet.

# Understanding Intermittent Fasting

Before you begin any diet or drastically change your eating pattern, it's always advisable to hunt the recommendation of a medical professional. This fact is often very actual if you've got an existing condition, as when there's fasting involved, it's going to interfere with your medication or health.

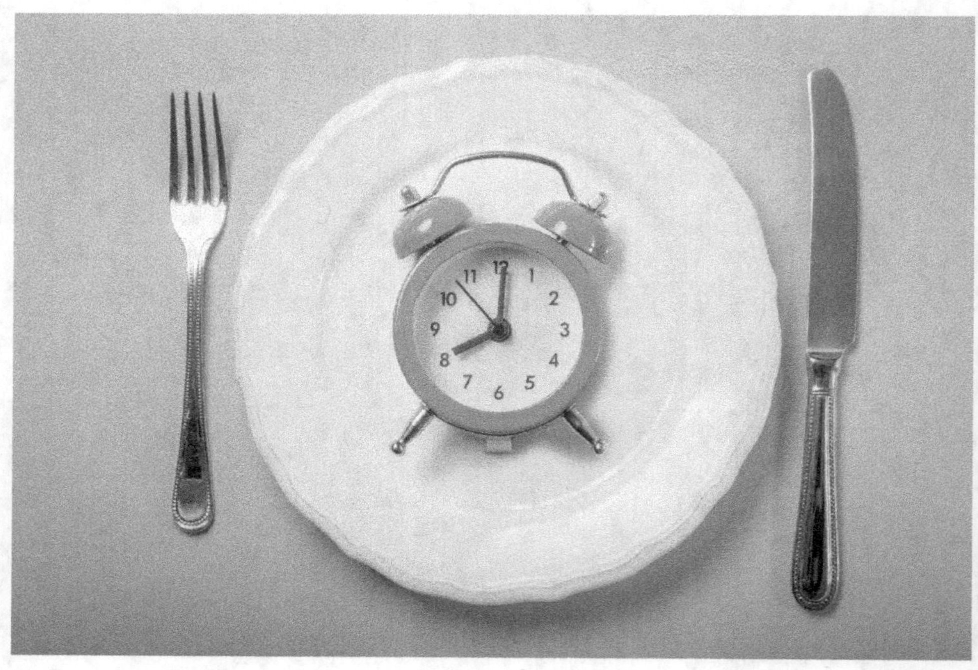

## What is the Intermittent Fasting Diet?

Intermittent fasting (IF) is when an individual refrains from eating at certain hours of the day. In the hours that the person isn't fasting, they eat a healthy, regimented diet. The intermittent fasting diet isn't such a lot of a diet but a lifestyle change.

Some of the more popular intermittent fasting methods are two to 3 days every week, alternate days, or daily in set hours. The thing about the intermittent fasting diet is that there's no need for counting calories, macronutrients, or lowering on certain foods.

There are no set rules aside from not eating specific set rules, and you'll eat what you wish in the time window in which you're not fasting. In the time once you are fasting, you'll drink water, tea, and occasional.

Intermittent fasting may be a diet that will be wont to reduce, enhance body composition, and reduce body fat. It's been known to possess tons of other health benefits, especially for ladies in life.

## History of Intermittent Fasting Diet

The father of recent medicine, Hippocrates of Cos, who lived between 460 BCE to 375 BCE, practiced fasting—fasting an ancient method of healing alongside apple vinegar. Plutarch was an Ancient Greek historian and writer; he also wrote about fasting instead of using medicine. Even Aristotle and his mentor Plato practiced and believed in fasting. (Fasting — A History Part 1, n.d.)

Fasting has been called the 'physician' in as all animals, also as humans, tend to show far away from food once they are sick. If you've got ever been ill, you'll know that the last item you think that of is food. It's as if fasting is ingrained into an individual's DNA, a natural instinctive reaction to sickness as old as time.

After an outsized meal, the body reduces blood flow to the brain because it pushes more blood to the gastrointestinal system to digest an excessive meal. Fasting was thought to enhance cognitive abilities by the traditional Greeks. But it had been not only the conventional Greeks and great philosophers that believed in fasting but the founding father of toxicology, Philip Paracelsus, did too.

Fasting has been used for several other reasons besides medical or losing weight also. It's also been used for spiritual purposes, religious purposes, purification, cleansing, and making statements for a cause.

Fasting has been around for several years and can be around for several more years as scientists have now begun to take an interest in its many benefits. Our ancient ancestors that were hunter-gatherers had to travel out trying to find food every day. Sometimes there was no food to be found, and then they might choose long periods without eating. As a result, the physical body evolved and adapted to be ready to go without food for days at a time.

The body functions better when it's been bereft of food for a few hours because it allows it to do some in-house cleaning.

## Why for ladies Over 50?

Women who approach post-menopause (and sometimes while early as pre-menopause) tend to start out accumulating belly fat. They're going to start noticing their metabolism gets slower. They'll also begin to feel aches and pains in their joints. Their sleep patterns start to urge entirely out of routine, leaving them feeling exhausted all the time. Then there's the load gain and a better risk of developing chronic diseases like cancer, diabetes, and a heart condition that would cause heart attacks.

There is also the danger of neurodegenerative diseases, stroke, and a continuing feeling of fatigue. Intermittent fasting has been known to reset an individual's internal balance. This manner, in turn, boosts their external appearance, energy levels, and cuts down on stress as they control their weight.

## Why Should Women Choose the Intermittent Fasting Diet?

Intermittent fasting has become a popular healthy lifestyle trend and permanently reason. It offers many health benefits also as it improves an individual's state of mind and encourages an all-round feeling of well-being.

# Types of Intermittent Fasting

There are different types or methods of intermittent fasting, which will be quite useful. The trick is checking out which is the best one for you that suits your needs and lifestyle.

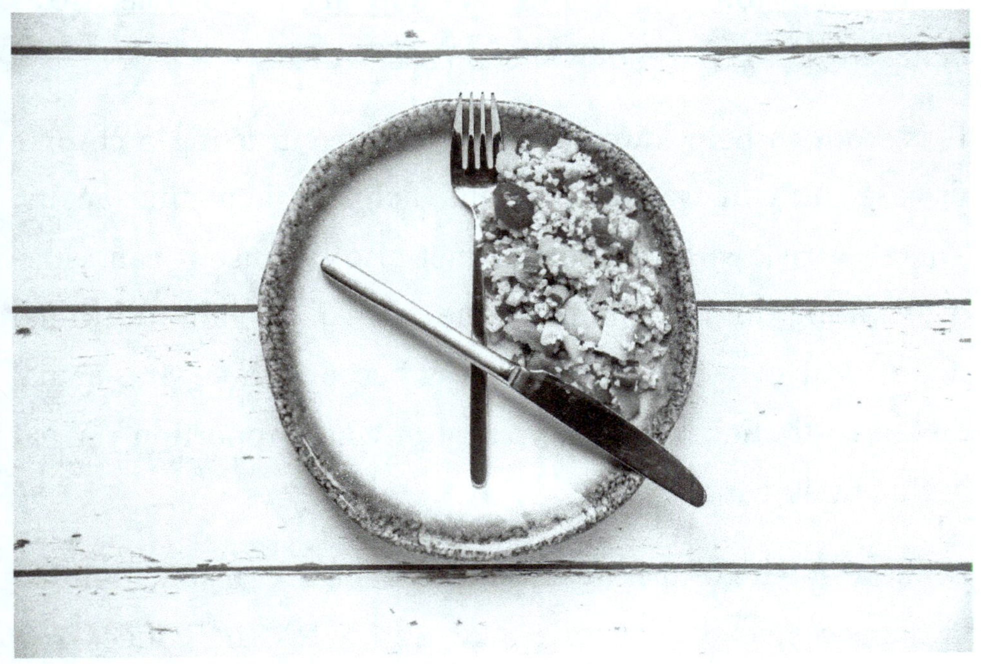

Fasting has periods where you do not eat then periods called cycles, patterns, or eating windows where an individual can eat. The following methods are the foremost effective for weight loss and are the most straightforward fasting cycles to follow.

# 16:8 Intermittent Fasting Method

The 16:8 intermittent fasting method is additionally referred to as the 8-hour diet as you fast for 16-hours each day and have an 8hour each day eating window. This method is employed by tons of celebrities and top business people also as being a well-liked trending diet on social media.

It is wont to help lower the danger of contracting a chronic disease, aids in weight loss, and helps with mental acuity. There's a risk with this sort of diet also because it can cause overheating in the limited time window if an individual doesn't eat correctly. Often, this is because there's no actual diet or restrictions on what you eat or what proportion you eat in that point window.

In the 16-hours of fasting, an individual can consume nothing but unsweetened beverages like water, tea, or coffee. You should not be consuming fizzy drinks, alcohol, or the other sweetened beverages because they're not healthy for you. They will also cause health problems due to what goes into those sorts of drinks.

In the 8-hour eating windows, an individual is liberal to eat what they please. most of the people who do the 16:8 fasting method find it easier to fast in the evening and thru breakfast subsequent day—leaving their 8-hour eating window to start at around noon or one o'clock. To urge the full benefits of an intermittent fasting diet, it is often beneficial to follow a diet plan that suits you. Tons of individuals will follow diets like the keto hotel plan, weight watchers, low-carb diets, etc.

The diet you select should be one that's beneficial to you and caters to your eating needs. What you are doing not want to do once you try to reap the advantages of intermittent fasting is to fill yourself abreast of empty carbs and sweets. Instead, make the foremost out of your eating window and eat healthily.

This intermittent fasting method isn't really for beginners, and if you'd wish to try it, you ought to try a modified version of it. Maybe attend 12:12, fast for 12 hours, and eat for 12 hours on a healthy eating plan. Only quickly with this method, no quite twice every week, once you first start with intermittent fasting.

## 5:2 Intermittent Fasting Method

The 5:2 diet is currently the foremost popular and practiced method of intermittent fasting and is understood because of the fast diet.

Michael Mosley, a British journalist who was diagnosed with type 2 diabetes in 2012, was the one who popularized this method. He managed to show his life around by losing 26.5 pounds in 12 weeks, which helped him get his type 2 diabetes check.

Throughout our lives, we are told that breakfast is the most important meal of the day. But who says it's to be eaten as soon as we rise or grab something as we leap out the door to start the day? Michael Mosley developed the 5:2 diet believing that an individual must give their body a rest from food.

The diet believes that when an individual goes without food for quite 10-hours, the body goes into harmful protein or balance. When this happens, the body starts to consume and obtain obviate old proteins and doesn't produce new ones. When the body doesn't receive enough or quality protein, it starts to finish what it can find and switches the body to cell repair mode.

An early supper and late breakfast are an honest thanks to allowing the body to clean itself out and repair what must be restored completely. On the 5:2 diet, an individual will eat a traditional healthy diet for five days of the week. The opposite two days, they're going to get on a calorie-restricted diet of 500 to 600 calories each day.

A person can choose the two days of the week that most accurately fits them as long as there's a minimum of one to 2 days in between fasting days. For example, fast on a Tuesday, eat the traditional number of calories required on Wednesday, then quickly on Thursday or Friday again. On fasting days, a lady should consume around 500 calories and check out to possess two small meals. The simplest eating plan is to maintain a late breakfast and an early supper to urge the most detailed results.

On eating days, a right, healthy diet should be followed to reduce and luxuriate in other health benefits of the diet alongside regular exercise.

## Alternate Day Fasting (ADF) Method

Alternate day fasting or ADF may be a fasting method done over 48 hours. An individual will fast for 36-hours (a day and a half) then eat normally for the 12-hour eating window. Of course, non-sweetened beverages like water, tea, and occasionally with no sugar are often drunk but nothing else in the 36-hours.

In the 12-hour eating window, people can eat a regular healthy diet or anything they need. There's a more popular version of this fasting method where people eat in a particular period and should consume up to 500 calories. Dr. Krista Varady brought out the "Every Other Day Diet" after studying the alternate-day fasting method.

Beginners to fasting methods find this intermittent fasting diet to be the simplest to take care of. Some studies show this method to be best for middle-aged women in losing and controlling their weight. Other studies have shown that it's going to be ready to reduce inflammation markers and belly fat, particularly those that are obese.

The alternate-day fasting method has shown to figure with or without a diet but is best when combined with regular exercise. To prevent or reduce compensatory hunger, the modified version of this fasting method is that the most recommended. Eating 500 calories each day at a particular time on fasting days with this method reduces hunger.

# Eat Stop Eat Intermittent Fasting Method

Brad Pilon developed this method of fasting after researching how it affects metabolism. The eat stop eat practice of fasting became famous after he wrote his popular book, Eat Stop Eat.

This fasting method takes an individual to possess two days every week once they fast. Lately must not be consecutive days, though, and will have a minimum of one to 2 eating days in between.

It sounds a touch painful as an individual has got to plan to fast for a full 24-hours. As an example, an individual could choose Monday and Thursday as their fasting days. This way ensures that there are two full days in between their fasting days. Choose time to start out fasting from Monday, which might be at 10 am, which provides you time to eat a simple breakfast before beginning your fast.

The fast would then end at 10 am on Tuesday, where an individual can enjoy a simple breakfast. They might eat their regular diet from 10 am Tuesday until 10 am Thursday once they start to fast again. The fast would stop at 10 am Friday, and for the remainder of the weekend, the person gets to eat their regular diet.

Although there are no actual dietary requirements for non-fasting days, it's highly recommended to follow a healthy diet. Or a minimum of making healthy food choices and choose foods that have slow-releasing carbs to eat just before starting the fast.

No matter what fasting method an individual chooses, it's imperative that they keep themselves well hydrated. Water is usually the most straightforward solution, although an unsweetened coffee or tea is often a pleasant change.

## The Warrior Diet

The warrior diet is sort of a strict intermittent fasting method because it follows a 20-hour restricted calorie intake diet and a 4-hour free diet window per day. This diet is predicated on the habits of human ancestors that might go hunting and gathering in the day. This meal plan can be for many days, starting in the early hours of the morning to return when the sun was taking place. It had been in these few hours before they slept that they might eat.

The warrior diet is predicated on fasting in the night and into the subsequent day until supper time. Then for 4-hours, it's recommended that an individual eats nutrient-dense foods, although there's no actual limit to what an individual can eat in this window. It is, however, advisable to eat the right foods like many whole-foods. Unprocessed foods are the foods to aim for on this diet, and therefore the excellent news is you don't need to count calories for 4-hours.

## One Meal each day (OMAD) Diet

This diet is not the fasting method recommended for beginners, and it shouldn't be taken lightly. Before this diet, an individual should first ask their medical advisor because it may be a 23:1 fasting method. This fact suggests that an individual cannot consume any calories for 23 hours of the day and only features a 1-hour eating window in which to eat.

Before trying this fasting method, an individual should learn the simplest times of day to eat. They ought to also know what the simplest foods are to eat in the 1-hour eating window. They ought to again only roll in the hay once or at the most twice every week unless they really know what they're doing.

It does, however, offer rapid weight loss and isn't too hard to follow. There's also no need for calories to be counted on the diet. In the 1-hour eating window, an individual can eat any food they need. Once more, healthy food choices are always the simplest option.

# The Benefits of Fasting for Women Over 50

Studies have shown that intermittent fasting could also be beneficial for postmenopausal women to maintain their weight. There are relatively few benefits to intermittent fasting for middle-aged women or women browsing menopause regardless of their age.

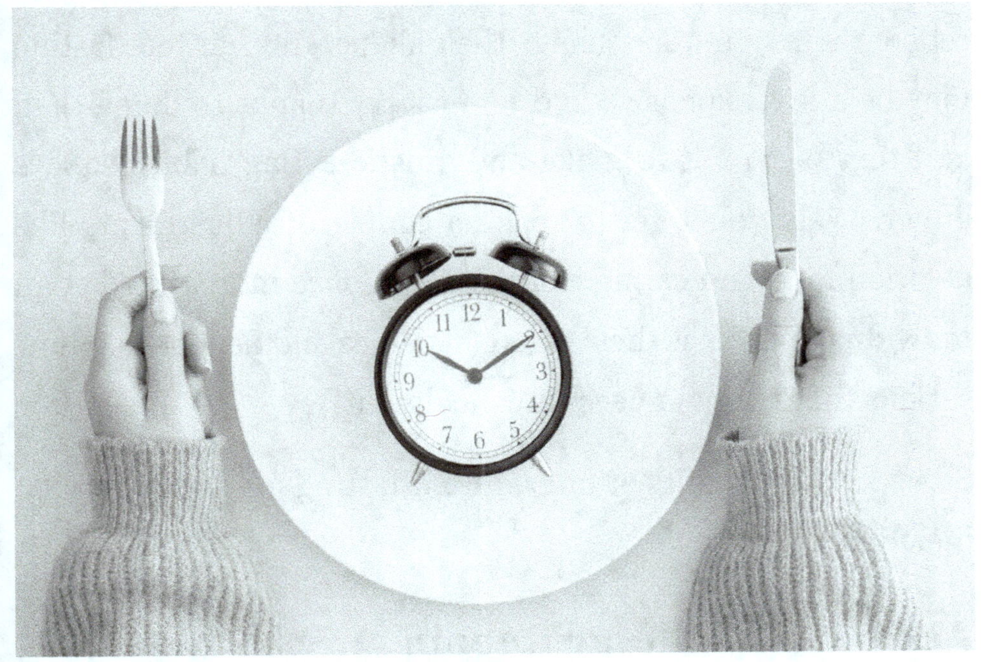

When women get to 50 and over, their skin will start to point out signs aged. They'll find their joints begin to ache for no reason, and suddenly belly fat accumulates as if you've got just born. There are numerous creams, diets, and exercises on the market to tighten the skin and check out to assist. The very fact is, they'll work to a particular point; on the other hand, the body hits a shelf, and zip seems to push an individual past it. This way boils up frustration, making women check out the more drastic and costly alternatives like surgery, which poses numerous more dangers and risks for ladies of fifty and over.

People don't get to go under the knife or starve themselves to reboot their system or change their shape. Intermittent fasting may be a less expensive and fewer risky thanks to doing that, and there's no got to make any drastic eating habit changes either. Well, you'll get to make a couple of adjustments like ablation food and eating healthier. But once more, the diet an individual follows is their personal choice and depends on how serious they're about becoming healthier.

Some health benefits of intermittent fasting for ladies over 50 include:

## Activating Cellular Repair

Fasting has been known to kick starter the body's natural cellular repair function, get and obviate mature cells, improve longevity, and improve hormone function, all things that tend to take a battering as people age. This manner will alleviate joint and muscle aches, also as lower back pain. The cells are being repaired, and the damage is undone, it helps with the skin's elasticity and health.

## Increase Cognitive Function and Protects the Brain from Damage

Intermittent fasting may increase the amount of a brain hormone referred to as a brain-derived neurotrophic factor (BDNF). It will equally guard the brain against damage sort of a stroke or Alzheimer's disease because it promotes new neuron growth. It also increases cognitive function and will effectively defend an individual against other neurodegenerative disorders also.

## Weight Loss

When people have belly fat, it can cause many health problems related to various diseases because it indicates an individual has visceral fat. Visceral fat is fat that goes deep into the abdominal surrounding the organs. Belly fat is tough to lose, especially for an aging woman. Intermittent fasting has been known to assist in reducing not only weight but inches of over five percent of body fat in around twenty-two to 25 weeks (Barna, 2019).

## Alleviates Oxidative Stress and Inflammation

Oxidative stress is when the body has an imbalance of antioxidants also as free radicals. This imbalance can cause both tissue and cell damage in overweight also as aging people. It also can cause various chronic illnesses like cancer, a heart condition, diabetes, and also has an impression on the signs of aging. Oxidative stress can trigger the inflammation that causes these diseases.

Intermittent fasting can provide your system with a reboot, helping to alleviate oxidative stress and inflammation in a middle-aged woman. It also significantly reduces the danger of oxidative stress and inflammation for those overweight or obese.

## Slow Down the Aging Process

As intermittent fasting gives both the metabolism and cellular repair a reboot, it offers the potential to hamper aging. It's going even to prolong an individual's lifespan by quite a few years, especially if following a nutritious diet and exercise regime alongside intermittent fasting.

# Balancing Hormones and Increasing Energy

The system is that the body's system that produces hormones. Hormones are potent chemicals that convey messages through the body to manage specific processes. Hormones are needed for growth, fertility, metabolism, the system, and their mood or behavior.

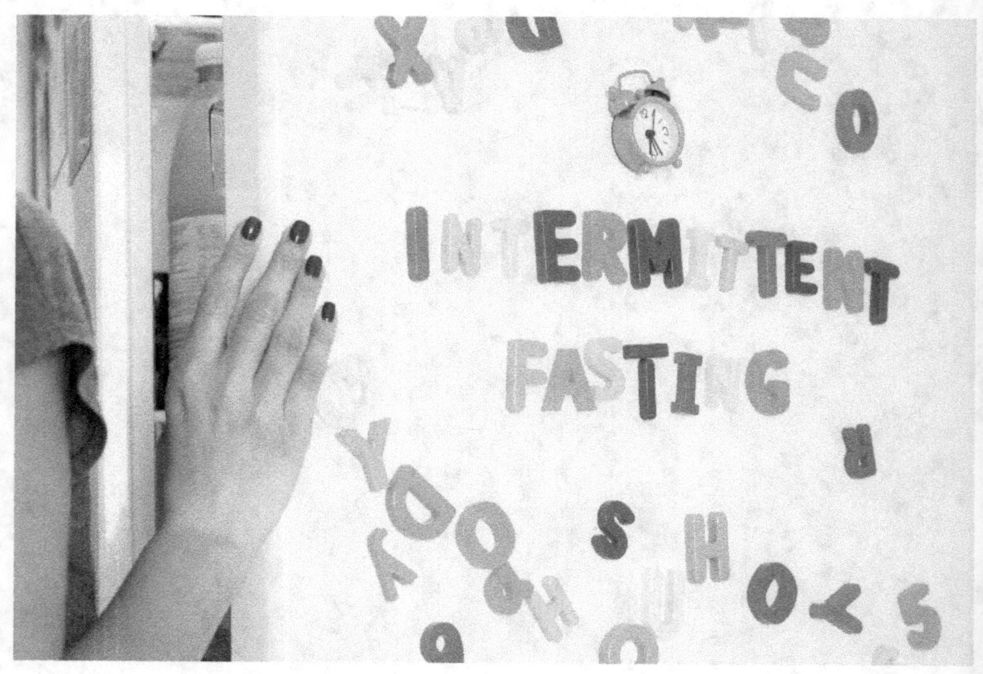

# Hormones

As we age, our hormones change, and our body produces more of some, less of others. Hormones are made following the person's stage of life. For instance, a teenager's hormones are produced to urge them through puberty—the subsequent stage of development for the physical body where hair starts to develop in strategic places. A woman's body changes and starts to urge ready for the next step to supply offspring.

In pregnancy, the body produces the human chorionic gonadotropin (HCG) hormone. Also, as human placental lactogen (HPL) hormone, estrogen, and progesterone. As most people know, women seem everywhere the place both physically and emotionally once they expect. Now you recognize why with of these extremely potent chemicals being produced.

Women undergo perimenopause, usually in their mid-forties. At this stage, the body's estrogen production starts to hamper until they are going through menopause. In menopause, the body stops releasing eggs, which suggests a lady is not any longer ready to reproduce.

Most women will undergo menopause between the ages of fifty-one to fifty-two. It can last anywhere from one to 3 years, and therefore the symptoms of menopause can include:

- The cycle has stopped for a year or more.
- Problems in sleeping.
- Bad nightly sweats, which will drench the person.
- Uncomfortably dry or itchy skin that seems like you've got a thousand ants crawling on you.
- Problems with urination, like releasing little drops when sneezing, problems urinating, and incontinence issues.
- Infections in the urinary tract or dryness, with a burning sensation
- A decreased libido and disinterest in intimacy
- Some women experience varying degrees of lethargy.
- Hot flashes that cause an individual to desire the doors of hell have opened ahead of them. These come on suddenly with no warning at any time or place in the day.

Some women will experience all of those symptoms, a number of them, et al. may get them more mildly or not in the least. Menopause and its symptoms are tons like being pregnant without parturition at the top. The hormones, or lack thereof, affect each woman differently. It wholly depends on how your body adjusts to the present introduces its lifecycle.

It is vital to undertake and balance your hormones. One hormone which increases when practicing intermittent fasting is that the somatotropin. As soon as an individual stops eating for long enough, the body starts to supply this hormone. The hormone sent bent repair tissue and is usually called the fountain of youth hormone thanks to its reparative qualities. While it doesn't do much to vary menopause, it'll help hamper the aging process and assist you in retaining muscle. It also helps with weight loss, and intermittent fasting has been shown to almost double this hormone in the body.

In menopause, two hormones that become imbalanced are melatonin and cortisol. These are the hormones that take to be in sync, as melatonin helps an individual sleep and luxuriate in good quality sleep. While cortisol is that the hormone that allows an individual to awaken, feel alert, and keep the mind clear. An imbalance of those two hormones is typically thanks to ill health, anxiety, stress, and menopause. Intermittent fasting alongside right nutrition may aid in the production and balance of those two hormones.

Homeostasis is that the term used for hormone balance, and it's vital for optimum health. To achieve success with an intermittent fasting program, you furthermore may need a nutritious diet. Once a lady reaches fifty, it's imperative to measure a healthy lifestyle to make sure you enjoy your time of life in peak make.

Women over fifty should strive to:

- Eat well but healthily and make smarter food choices.
- Fast in their temperature and make it a neighborhood of their life.
- Take supplements to make sure they're getting enough vitamins and minerals.
- Take care of their skin by implementing the right treatments in or out of the sun.
- Wear protection in the heat when outside. Wear a hat to hide your face and neck. Wear sun protection, although an honest quarter-hour of direct sunlight will increase vitamin D.
- Exercise a minimum of two to 3 times every week, more if you're ready to.
- Most importantly, drink a lot of water.

# Energy

Hormones can equally affect an individual's energy levels. In menstrual cycles, energy levels are known to spike and rise thanks to increased levels of estrogen. But after the process, the amount of estrogen drops quite drastically, causing lethargy. As women reach menopause and estrogen levels start to drop, women feel less energetic and very tired.

Another hormonal culprit that contributes to a menopausal woman's lack of energy is progesterone. This hormone declines with age and is one among the explanations middle-aged women have problems sleeping. Progesterone is employed to induce ovulation in younger ladies, but it also promotes sleep. A lady's browsing time of life does not need ovulation, so her body doesn't produce the maximum amount because it won't happen.

Although they are doing not produce it in the amounts a person does, an adult female body also has testosterone. Testosterone performs a big part in the production of red blood cells in the body. Red blood cells are the cells that transport oxygen around the body, which may be a much-needed component in the promotion of energy. Like many other hormones, menopause limits the assembly of testosterone also.

High-stress levels will cause a rise in cortisol, which, as discussed in the previous section, you'll know keeps an individual awake. This fact affects sleep patterns, which is merely another added factor causing a scarcity of energy thanks to feeling tired. It'll even have an impression on a woman's mood and leave them feeling horrible.

There are ways to extend energy levels, but the primary step to take is to live your hormone levels. This fact will be done by your medical advisor, a registered clinic, or there are home tests you'll patronize the pharmacy. Ask a pharmacist what the most specific and most reliable brands are. Once you recognize what you're handling, there are a couple of methods you'll attempt to increase energy levels.

- Never try hormone replacements or balancing hormones without the recommendation of a medical professional. If you're not on any medication or have any pre-existing medical conditions, you'll try one among the following tips:

- Ask your doctor, nutritionist, or pharmacist to recommend an honest quality multi-vitamin. Confirm you fall under a routine of taking them.

- Slowly change your diet to at least one that gives more nutrition and agrees together with your system. As you age, you'll find foods that you simply may not be ready to eat.

- Find a quiet time to take ten to fifteen minutes to meditate, clear your mind, and learn the art of breathing.

- Tibetan monks have practiced anapanasati, which is mindfulness through breathing.

- Get enough good quality sleep. You'll get to make some adjustments to your bedroom. Confirm your pillow is supporting your head, which your mattress is doing an equivalent for your body. Take all electronics out of your room; if you employ your mobile for an alarm, confirm it goes into sleep mode. Rather than a TV, make space for a chair to twist up in and skim. Reading before bed may be an excellent way to unwind and slip into another world to clear your mind. Try not to take naps in the day.

- Get in some exercise a minimum of once each day, twice if you'll manage it. It doesn't mean you've got to travel running a marathon or do the Tour de France. Choose a walk, do some gardening, or take a mild bike ride and appearance at the scenery.
- Find a replacement hobby or take up an old one you had forgotten. If you engage your mind, you'll automatically gear your body up for action.
- There are supplements and specific foods to boost your energy naturally. Whatever you are doing, don't try highly caffeinated drinks or other such sorts of energy boosters you discover in a supermarket.

By now, you'll know a subsequent little bit of advice goes to be — drink much water. It's an excellent cure for an entire lot of things, including lethargy. If you would like to urge a touch extra boost, try using an icepack on your vagus in your neck for a moment at a time.

# Getting Started

There are a couple of things that an individual must know before diving in and proceed with intermittent fasting. One of the primary things is that it's going to be a simple idea to possess a general checkup and chat together with your medical man before you begin fasting. A couple of blood workups or an entire physical can establish a baseline from which to start. You'll be ready to find out a perfect fasting plan also as an appropriate diet that has any supplements, micronutrients, and macronutrients you'll take.

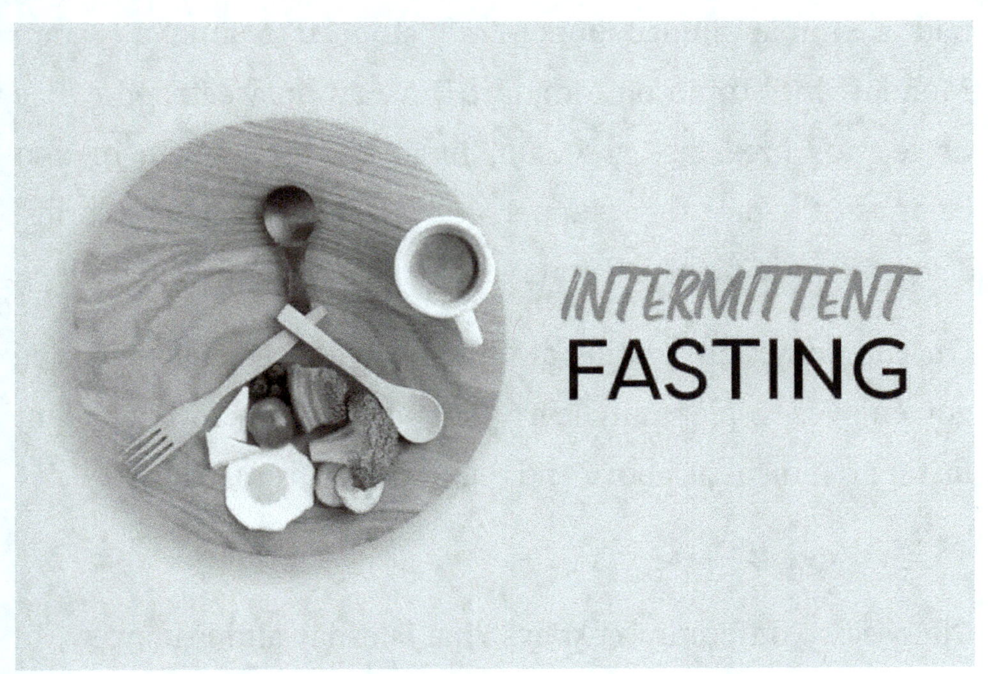

# Fasting Plan for 5:2 Combined With 12:12

When you are first starting, you'll want to possess a four-week cycle.

For instance:

### Week 1

Fasting Days are Monday and Thursday. Fasting time is 12 hours, with only non-caloric beverages and 12 hours where you'll eat a maximum of 500 calories per day (two meals).

For Monday, start fasting at 9 pm on Sunday after you've got had a simple filling supper and stopped fasting at 9 am Monday until 9 pm on Monday. Have an unsweetened coffee or tea for breakfast at 9 am, lunch to a complete of 250 calories at 1 pm, then supper at 7 or 8 pm of 250 calories. Tuesday morning, you'll start eating normally for the day.

On Thursday, start fasting at 9 pm on Wednesday after you've got enjoyed a pleasant hearty supper. Follow an equivalent fasting regiment as above and regularly eat from Friday.

### Week 2

Choose two different weekdays, like Tuesday and Friday.

For Tuesday, start fasting at 9 pm on Monday after a hearty supper and follow an equivalent method as Monday/Thursday above. Eat regularly on Wednesday and Thursday for the day.

Friday, you'll start to fast at 9 pm on Thursday once more after a simple supper. Follow an equivalent method as Monday, Thursday, and Tuesday above. You'll start eating normally on Saturday morning again.

### Week 3

Choose another two different days of the week, like Wednesday and Saturday. Most of the people balk at having to fast on a Saturday, but it takes great discipline, and you'll always keep Sundays as your non-fasting day.

Wednesday, you'll start fasting at 9 pm on Tuesday, following an equivalent method because the days above, to start out eating normally again on Thursday morning.

Saturday, you'll start fasting at 9 pm on Friday. Follow an equivalent method because of the days above, where you'll begin to eat on Sunday morning regularly.

**Week 4**

On week four, you ought to not fast but instead eat normally a day then start the fasting week over the subsequent week again.

## Non-Fasting Days

As with the methods above, the times where you're not fasting, you'll eat a traditional diet. Although there are not any specific diet rules to follow once you are on eating days or eating windows, it's highly recommended to follow a natural, nutritious diet. After all, you would like to reap the full benefits of this manner of life, see results, and feel better. You'll still reap several advantages if you eat what you wish.

To make life even easier for you, determine what your recommended daily calorie intake is. This fact is often determined by your height, bone structure, muscle mass, the way you carry your fat deposits, also as your age and gender.

Once you've got that, you simply can determine what your weekly calorie intake should be.

For example, a mean woman needs 2,000 calories each day to take care of a healthy weight, and fasting days are 25% of the two,000 calories (500 calories).

2,000 calories per day x 7 days = 14,000 calories every week

500 calories per day x 2 fasting days = 1,000 calories every week for fasting days

14,000 calories per week - 1,000 calories every week for fasting days = 13,000 calories every week

13,000 calories per week / 5 non-fasting days per week = 2,800 calories per non-fasting days

You should eat in your weekly calorie amount and not re-evaluate. It's better to undertake and keep your calories either at 14,000 calories per week and a couple of 000 calories per non-fasting days. To boost your metabolism, try calorie cycling together with your non-fasting days. Calories cycling is once you eat 2,000 calories at some point, 1,000 calories another day, then 2,250 calories on another day, non-fasting days that's.

When calorie cycling, you want not to exceed your weekly calorie amount. If you begin your calorie cycling on a Monday, then you simply have until that Sunday night to eat your weekly amount. The subsequent Monday, your calories set back to 14,000 calories.

Choose a natural diet or make healthy food choices if you're getting to continue together with your regular eating patterns. You are doing not need to make drastic changes, but rather than reaching for a treat filled with empty carbs, go for one that has some nutritional value. They're not loaded with anything artificial and taste even as good. Before you recognize it, you'll have retrained your mind to instead choose the healthier alternative to your favorite foods or beverages.

# 7-Day Intermittent Food Plan

One way to keep on a healthy diet is to plan your meals for the week ahead of time. That way, you can get the shopping done more efficiently precisely, as you know what you want to buy. It is also a great way to budget. You can prepare some meals in advance to save time, and you keep yourself on a healthy eating track.

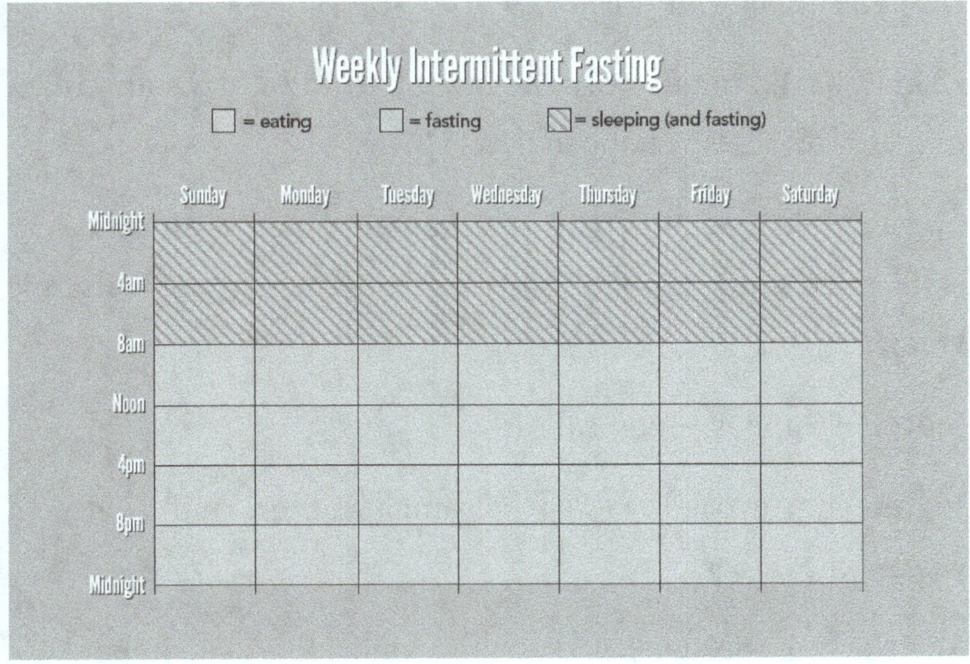


The following 7-day meal plan is an example of what you can eat on your fasting days and non-fasting days. Remember to stay in your weekly calorie limit and go for healthier choices.

For instance, instead of taking full-fat vanilla ice cream, choose low-fat and sugar-free. Choose raw almonds instead of salted ones and so on.

## Day 1 — Fasting Day 500 Calorie Allowance

9:00 AM Breakfast — 0 calories

A cup of unsweetened coffee or tea.

1:00 PM Lunch — 231 calories

1 small baked potato with ½ tsp butter and 2 tsp sour cream topped with ½ tsp chopped fresh chives.

Garden salad with ¼ cup of iceberg lettuce, 1 small celery stalk, 1 medium tomato, and drizzle with 1 tsp of balsamic vinegar.

8:00 PM Supper — 223 calories

¼ medium avocado, 1 tsp balsamic vinegar, and 1 slice of whole-wheat toast.

Add the same garden salad as above and add ¼ cucumber.

# Day 2 — Non-Fasting Day 2 000 Calorie Allowance

9:00 AM Breakfast — 412 calories

2-egg omelet with 2 tbsp cheddar cheese, 1 tsp chopped spring onion, and 1 tbsp chopped button mushrooms.

1 slice of whole-wheat toast with 1 tsp butter.

11:00 AM Snack — 166 calories

½ cup low-fat Greek yogurt, with 1 tsp organic honey, and ½ cup halved strawberries (fresh or frozen).

1:00 PM Lunch — 491 calories

6 shoots of grilled asparagus and 1 salmon fillet with lemon butter and dill sauce.

1 bowl of Caesar salad with dressing and croutons

1 cup sugar-free butterscotch pudding.

3:00 PM Snack — 150 calories

2 tbsp feta cheese, ¼ cup of olives, 2 tbsp low-fat cottage cheese, 3 small breadsticks.

8:00 PM Supper — 698 calories

1 flame-grilled cheeseburger with a 1 cup of oven-baked fries with low-sodium salt to taste.

1 cup fat-free vanilla ice cream with ½ cup blueberries (fresh or frozen) and ½ cup raspberries (fresh or frozen)

10:00 PM Snack — 66 calories

½ cup of blackberries and 5 raw almonds.

## Day 3 — Non-Fasting Day 2 000 Calorie Allowance

9:00 AM Breakfast — 492 calories

1 cup of organic rolled oats cooked, add ¼ cup unsweetened almond milk, 1 sliced banana, ¼ cup mixed berries(frozen or fresh), 3 tsp organic honey, and 2 tbsp raw almond slices.

11:00 AM Snack — 128 calories

½ cup low-fat plain chunky cottage cheese with 2 tsp organic honey, 2 tbsp blackberries, 2 tbsp raspberries, and 1 tbsp raw cashew nuts. The berries can be either fresh or frozen, and the cashews should be unsalted.

1:00 PM Lunch — 393 calories

2 slices whole-wheat bread, 2 tsp butter, 2 pieces of turkey, 2 tbsp shredded cheddar cheese, 1 tsp low-fat mayonnaise, ¼ sliced tomato, 2 lettuce leaves, and 2 tsp alfalfa sprouts. Make a delicious filling sandwich.

Slice up ¼ apple, 5 grapes, 2 tbsp low-fat Greek yogurt, 1 tsp organic honey, ¼ tsp ground cinnamon, and ¼ tsp cayenne pepper for extra zing (optional). Mix in a dessert bowl for a treat after your sandwich.

3:00 PM Snack — 173 calories

2 plain, no salt added rice cakes, 2 tbsp plain low-fat cream cheese, 1 tsp organic honey, and ¼ tsp ground cinnamon. Spread a bit of cream cheese on each rice cake, drizzle with a bit of the honey and add a dash of ground cinnamon on top.

8:00 PM Supper — 692 calories

1 lean grilled chicken breast (spiced as you take and cut into chunks), ¼ cup cooked wild rice, ¼ tsp ground ginger, ¼ tsp ground cinnamon, ¼ cup cooked garden peas, 3 tbsp diced spring onions, and 1 tbsp low-fat mayonnaise. Serve the chicken and rice warm, add the rest of the ingredients after you have mixed up the rice and chicken in a dinner bowl.

1 cup fat-free vanilla ice cream with ½ cup fresh, halved strawberries, 1 diced kiwi, and ½ cup diced fresh mango. Drizzle with 1 tsp organic honey and sprinkle with all-spice as well as chopped raw cashews.

10:00 PM Snack — 139 calories 20 raw almonds.

## Day 4 — Fasting Day 500 Calorie Allowance

9:00 AM Breakfast — 0 calories

A cup of unsweetened coffee or tea.

1:00 PM Lunch — 269 calories

2 large bell peppers (cut in half), 3 tbsp cooked wild rice, 1 tsp capers, ½ oz lean grilled chicken breasts shredded, and 2 tsp reduced-fat mayonnaise. Divide filling and stuff evenly between each bell pepper half. 8:00 PM Supper — 224 calories

1 grilled sole fillet with 1 tsp garlic butter.

Garden salad with 1 cup of iceberg lettuce, 1 medium tomato chopped, ¼ cucumber, 1 tbsp spring onions, ½ cup button mushrooms, 2 tbsp yellow bell pepper, and 1 tbsp organic balsamic vinegar.

# Day 5 — Non-Fasting Day 2 000 Calorie Allowance

9:00 AM Breakfast — 528 calories

2 eggs scrambled with 2 tbsp shredded cheddar cheese, 2 tbsp shredded mozzarella cheese, and 1 tsp chopped spring onion.

2 slice of whole-wheat toast with 1 tsp butter

1 medium apple

11:00 AM Snack — 173 calories

¼ cup regular trail mix

1:00 PM Lunch — 523 calories

1 low-carb whole wheat tortilla stuffed with shredded lettuce, ½ chopped tomato, 4 cooked and crumbled pieces of bacon, ¼ chopped avocado, 2 chopped pickles, 1 tbsp low-fat mayonnaise.

1 medium-sized peach

3:00 PM Snack — 118 calories

Mixed berry smoothie, 2 tbsp blueberries, 2 tbsp blackberries, 2 tbsp raspberries, ¼ cup organic low-fat unsweetened almond milk, and 4 tbsp low-fat Greek yogurt.

8:00 PM Supper — 683 calories

1 large whole wheat tortilla, spread the base with 2 tsp organic unsweetened tomato paste, top with 4 tbsp shredded mozzarella cheese, top with 1 cup cooked shredded chicken breast, ½ thinly sliced tomato. Then top with ½ tsp capers, 1 tbsp pitted black olives, drizzle with 2 tbsp fruit chutney, and last sprinkle 4 tbsp shredded cheddar cheese over the top. Put the tortilla pizza into a preheated oven and cook for around 18-20 minutes or until brown.

1 large banana sliced lengthwise, ¼ cup fat-free vanilla ice cream, ¼ mixed berries fresh or frozen, 1 large plum cut into chunks, ½ pear cut into pieces, and 1 tbsp unsweetened desiccated coconut. Make the ingredients into a banana boat and top with the desiccated coconut.

10:00 PM Snack — 150 calories 4 pieces of dark chocolate.

# Day 6 — Non-Fasting Day 2 000 Calorie Allowance

9:00 AM Breakfast — 348 calories

In a dessert bowl or parfait glass, add 4 tbsp organic sugar-free granola, top with 5 tbsp fat-free strawberry yogurt, top with 1 tbsp blackberries, 1 tbsp raspberries, 1 tbsp blueberries. Then top with 4 tbsp fat-free plain Greek yogurt, drizzle over 1 tsp of organic honey, sprinkle 1 tsp of toasted almond flakes, 1 tsp chia seeds, and 1 tsp unsweetened desiccated coconut.

11:00 AM Snack — 183 calories

1 peanut butter protein bar

2 small apricots

1:00 PM Lunch — 413 calories

1 bowl of chicken Caesar salad with dressing and croutons

1 large banana

1 cup of grapes

3:00 PM Snack — 184 calories

¼ cup of olives

½ cup of fresh cauliflower divided into florets

½ cup carrots cut into sticks

½ cup cucumber cut into sticks

¼ cup tzatziki

8:00 PM Supper — 653 calories

1 roasted chicken breast, 4 roast potatoes, ½ cup cooked corn, ½ cup cooked carrots, and ½ cup cooked peas

1 cup fat-free vanilla ice cream topped with 2 tsp organic cocoa powder, 2 tsp organic honey, and 1 tbsp raw unsalted cashews.

10:00 PM Snack — 150 calories 4 pieces of dark chocolate.

## Day 7 — Non-Fasting Day 2 000 Calorie Allowance

9:00 AM Breakfast — 399 calories

1 chopped apple, 1 chopped plum, ¼ papaya chopped, 1 banana sliced, ¼ cup fresh halved strawberries, ¼ cup blueberries, 1 tsp sunflower seeds, and 2 tbsp low-fat vanilla Greek yogurt.

1 glass unsweetened organic light coconut milk.

11:00 AM Snack — 150 calories 4 pieces of dark chocolate.

1:00 PM Lunch — 657 calories

1 bowl of chicken soup with 2 slices of whole-wheat toast and 2 tsp butter.

1 small green salad.

1 cup sugar-free butterscotch pudding with ½ cup of fat-free vanilla ice cream.

3:00 PM Snack — 228 calories

3 graham crackers with 1 tbsp Nutella.

8:00 PM Supper — 795 calories

1 grilled chicken burger with a 1 cup of oven-baked fries with low-sodium salt to taste.

1 small green salad.

1 slice of cheesecake, 1 tbsp low-fat unsweetened whipped cream, and 1 tsp macadamia nuts.

10:00 PM Snack 104 calories

½ cup of blackberries, ½ cup of raspberries, and ¼ of blueberries.

Total calories for the week = 11 386 calories, which are 2614 calories less than the weekly total.

As you can see, by the meal plan that you can eat great meals with dessert and still come in well under the recommended calorie intake for the week. All you have to do is make healthier food choices when shopping, going out to eat, or at a dinner party.

# Ideas for Healthy Eating

Eating significantly healthy, complements your new fasting lifestyle. But you furthermore may need to make sure that you're getting enough nutrition in your diets also.

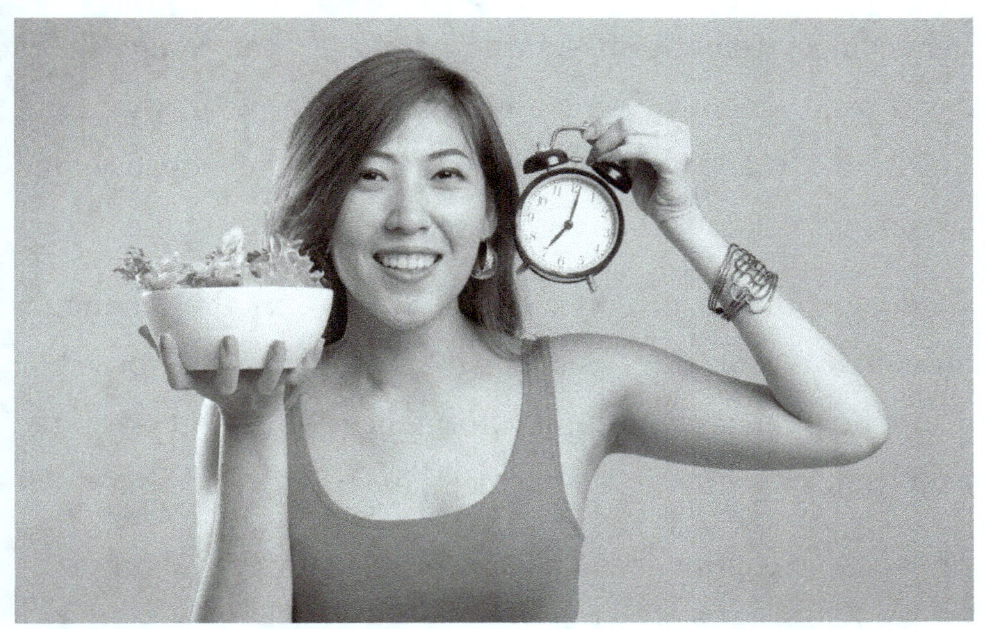

## Eating Nutritiously for ladies Aged 50 and Over

As a woman, your body has specific nutrient needs that have got to be fulfilled to take care of healthiness. You'll get a natural source of those vitamins and minerals through supplements, but nothing beats the more natural way through food sources.

A lot of girls tend to come short of getting into their daily nutritional requirements. Getting into the right dietary requirements also can improve your energy levels, mood, and help control weight gain. As your body ages, you would like to assist and keep it functioning correctly with the right nutrition. It also can assist you through menopause and beyond to make sure you've got an honest quality of life.

When you are fasting, it's crucial to urge in the maximum amount of your daily recommended nutrients as possible. These help the body to supply hormones and energy, keep the skin healthy, promote healthy teeth, hair, nails, and bones.

The RDA (recommended daily allowance) of the vital nutrients for ladies 50 and over are:

## Calcium - 1,200 mg per day

Calcium is required for strong bones and healthy teeth. It also aids in regulating the heartbeat, and a deficiency of it affects your teeth, bones, and mood. Not getting enough calcium can cause osteoporosis. This fact is often because the body will start to take calcium from the bones to assist normal cell function.

Foods that are high in calcium include:

- Low-fat, plain Greek yogurt
- Full-cream milk, non-fat milk, 2% milk, or reduced-fat milk (find a spread fortified with vitamin D)
- Cheeses: cheddar, mozzarella, cheese, feta, parmesan, and pot cheese
- Tofu that states it's made with calcium sulfate
- Nut milk
- Soy milk
- Kale, broccoli, Chinese cabbage, and turnips
- Salmon, shrimp, and sardines
- Oranges and figs
- Fortified cereals
- Baked beans or most canned beans

**Iron - 8 mg per day**

Iron is a crucial nutrient the body must maintain healthy hair, skin, nails, and hemoglobin. Hemoglobin is the compound that oxygenates the blood. A deficiency of iron can cause anemia, which may cause an individual to feel weak and lethargic.

Foods that are high in iron include:

- Raisins
- Bell peppers
- Leafy green vegetables like spinach
- Eggs (boiled)
- Cashew nuts
- Potatoes
- Broccoli, peas, and green beans
- Tuna, oysters, sardines, and muscles
- Turkey and chicken
- Liver
- Beef
- Kidney beans, white beans, lentils, and chickpeas
- Tomatoes
- Bread
- Tofu
- Nuts and seeds
- Some edible fruit
- Breakfast cereals

- Dark chocolate

**Magnesium - 400 mg per day**

Magnesium may be a nutrient needed to assist and keep bones and teeth healthy. It also aids in ensuring that your nervous systems and muscles work correctly. Magnesium is required to support the right insulin levels, even as heart health.

Foods that are high in magnesium include:

- Avocado
- Dark chocolate
- Nuts and seeds
- Most fruit, especially raspberries, bananas, and figs
- Chickpeas, kidney beans, baked beans, and black beans
- Peas, broccoli, cabbage, green beans, asparagus, and artichokes
- Tuna, mackerel, salmon, and sardines
- Bread, oats, and rice
- Cacao (raw organic)
- Tofu
- Leafy green vegetables like kale, spinach, and lettuce

**Vitamin A - 700 mcg per day**

Vitamin A may be a multifunctional vitamin that plays a crucial role keep the interior organs, kidney, lungs, and heart working as they ought to. It also supports the system, reproduction system, and eyesight.

Foods that are high in vitamin A include:

- Liver
- Cod liver oil
- Tuna, mackerel, trout, and salmon
- Butter
- Cheese, especially chevre
- Boiled egg
- Sweet potato, butternut squash, and carrots
- Spinach, broccoli, bell pepper, and lettuce
- Melons and grapefruit

**Vitamin C - 75 mg per day**

Vitamin C is another vitamin that plays an essential part in many operations in the body. It aids the system, repairs cell tissue, is significant for growth and normal development. It helps the body absorb iron and sees to the care of bones, teeth, and muscles. It plays a crucial part in skin health because it helps with the creation of collagen also because of the healing of wounds.

Foods that are high in vitamin C include:

- Oranges
- Clementines
- Grapefruit
- Kiwis
- Pineapple Apricots
- Mangos
- Guava
- Strawberries Papaya
- Bell peppers
- Kale
- Brussel Sprouts
- Broccoli
- Cauliflower
- Yellow melons
- Chilis

**Vitamin B-6 - 1.5 mg Per Day**

The B vitamins work together to assist with the metabolism, growth, liver function, and therefore the creation of blood cells. Vitamin B-6 is employed in the production of the sleep hormone, melatonin.

Foods that are high in vitamin B-6 include:

- Peanuts
- Eggs
- Fish
- Poultry
- Pork
- Bread
- Wholegrain cereals
- Fortified cereals
- Potatoes
- Milk
- Vegetables
- Soya beans

**Vitamin B-9 (Folate) - 400 mcg per day**

The B vitamins work together and with other nutrients to make red blood cells. Folate is additionally a crucial vitamin that ensures iron is correctly absorbed and utilized in the body. Vitamin B-9 is employed to assist in regulating the amino alkanoic acid homocysteine blood levels.

Foods that are high in vitamin B-9 include:

- Seafood
- Eggs
- Most fresh fruit
- Most fresh fruit juices
- Liver
- Peanuts
- Beans
- Whole grains
- Sunflower seeds
- Broccoli
- Turnip greens
- Asparagus
- Spinach
- Brussel sprouts
- Lettuce
- Green beans

**Vitamin B-12 - 2.4 mcg per day**

Vitamin B-12 helps to stop anemia because it aids the body in inadequately absorbing and utilizing iron. It helps in the production of DNA and regulates the blood cells and, therefore, the system.

Foods that are high in vitamin B-12 include:

- Kidneys
- Liver
- Beef
- Other edible animal organs
- Sardines, tuna, trout, herring, and salmon
- Clams, shrimp, mussels, crab, and oysters
- Fortified dairy products
- Eggs
- Ham and pork
- Chicken and turkey
- Plain Greek yogurt
- Cottage, cheese, ricotta, and mozzarella cheese Nutritional yeast

**Vitamin D - 15 mg per day**

One of the most functions of vitamin D helps the body to soak up calcium to make sure healthy bones and teeth. It also supports the system, promotes good skin health, may reduce depression, and it can increase weight loss.

Foods that are high in vitamin D include:

- Some nuts and seeds contain vitamin D
- Beef liver
- Egg yolk
- Tuna, salmon, and mackerel
- Fortified dairy products
- Fortified cereals

**Vitamin E — 15 mcg per day**

Vitamin E is just like the soldier's nutrient of the body. It's wont to help repel harmful bacteria, protects cells against damage, it's an antioxidant, and it boosts the system . vitamin E is additionally vital for firmer, younger-looking skin.

Foods that are high in vitamin E include:

- Almonds
- Pine nuts
- Peanuts
- Seeds like sunflower seeds
- Spinach
- Broccoli
- Butternut squash

- Avocado
- Kiwi
- Mangos
- Shrimp
- Lobster
- Trout, salmon, and cod
- Goose
- Olive oil

**Vitamin K - 90 mcg per day**

Vitamin K is a crucial nutrient that helps with bone metabolism and controls calcium levels in the blood. It's also a significant agent that helps in the production of prothrombin, which may be a protein utilized in blood coagulation.

Foods that are high in vitamin K include:

- Swiss chard
- Mustard greens
- Kale
- Spinach and broccoli
- Liver
- Prunes
- Kiwi

- Hard cheeses
- Avocado
- Green peas Cabbage
- Broccoli

## Healthy Eating Ideas

While fasting, you ought to attempt to eat breakfast later in the day if you're fasting through the night.

Suppose you've got chosen the fasting hotel plan that permits an individual to consume a limited number of calories per day, attempt to eat only two meals each day — lunch and supper. But if you want to eat breakfast, then make it a smaller one, take no quite 50 calories from lunch and 70 from dinner. It's better to stay the evening meal lighter than your afternoon one as you would like the energy from lunch to urge you thru the whole day.

### Fasting Plan Without Calorie Restriction

Drink tons of water that can be infused with mint. Mint keeps you alert and provides the water a pleasant flavor, but you can't put anything to sweeten it in the water.

Drink tea or coffee with no sweeteners, sugar, cream, or flavors. You'll put a touch of cayenne pepper in the drink to offer it a kick and help burn calories.

**Fasting Plan With Calorie Restriction**

Fasting day with calorie-restrictive eating windows is predicated on 500 calories each day.

The breakdown for 500 calories fasting day restriction would be:

With small breakfast

- Breakfast = 130 calories
- Lunch = 200 calories
- Dinner = 170 calories

Lunch and dinner only

- Breakfast = 0 calories
- Lunch = 250 calories
- Dinner = 250 calories

## Normal Eating (Non-Fasting) Days or Eating Window Food Ideas

Non-fasting day food ideas have supported a mean of two,000 calories each day. If you're eager to reduce, you ought to check out cutting that right down to around 1,500 calories each day.

The breakdown for the typical day eating at 2,000 calories each day (14,000 calories per week) would be:

- Breakfast = 500 calories
- Mid-morning snack = 200 calories
- Lunch = 500 calories
- Mid-afternoon snack = 200 calories
- Dinner = 500 calories
- Light before bed snack = 100 calories

Always drink a glass of warm water before getting to sleep. Warm water will help debar night cramps, relieve pain, and helps to rid the body of unwanted toxins. This fact is often because warm water is excellent for circulation. It'll also keep you hydrated in the long hours of the night, which successively will assist you to have an honest quality night's rest.

# Healthy Breakfast Ideas

The following are a couple of quick and straightforward healthy breakfast ideas to assist kick-starter your morning.

## Fasting Without Limited Calories

This method is usually done in the evening and into mid-morning the subsequent day. If it does span each day, there are nonfasting windows where an individual can eat normally. See the non-fasting healthy ideas for ordinary eating day breakfast ideas.

## Fasting With Limited Calories (100 to 130 Calories)

The following recipes are 130 calories and under.

Blueberry Mango Yogurt - 97 Calories

- 1 small mango chopped
- 1 oz blueberries (fresh or frozen)
- 4 tbsp non-fat plain Greek yogurt
- dash of ground cinnamon

Spoon the yogurt into a parfait glass or dessert bowl, add the chopped mango and blueberries. Add a dash of cinnamon for taste and to add a bit of sweetness.

Egg White Mushroom Scramble - 93 Calories

- 3 tbsp fresh button mushrooms chopped
- 3 fresh egg whites
- 1 tsp coconut oil to cook with
- low-sodium salt and black pepper to taste

Heat the coconut oil in a skillet over medium heat. Add the egg whites and mushrooms, stir into a scramble, then serve hot.

Cold Watermelon, Grapefruit, Kiwi, and Pomegranate Cup - 100 Calories

- 1 tbsp pomegranate seeds
- ½ small chopped kiwi fruit
- ½ small grapefruit
- ¼ cup iced, cubed fresh watermelon

Freeze the watermelon the night before. Add all the chopped fruit to a cereal or dessert bowl and enjoy a fresh fruit salad for breakfast.

Almonds, Banana, and Honey - 129 Calories

- 1 small banana sliced
- 1 tbsp organic coconut flakes
- 1 tsp organic honey

Slice the banana and add it to a cereal or dessert bowl. Drizzle with organic honey, sprinkle over the coconut flakes, and enjoy.

Mixed Berry Coconut Smoothie - 121 Calories

- 3 tbsp blueberries
- 3 tbsp raspberries
- 3 tbsp blackberries
- 2 tsp shredded unsweetened coconut shreds
- ¼ cup unsweetened coconut water
- ½ cup still mineral water
- 1 tsp organic honey
- dash of cinnamon to taste

Add all the ingredients into a blender. Blend until the smoothie is thick and smooth. Add to a glass and drink or pack it in a container to take with you.

Healthy Breakfast Ideas for Normal Eating Days (500 Calories and Under)

These easy breakfast recipes are filled with nutrients and are only 500 calories or less. Boiled Egg, Avocado, and Red Radish,

Rocket Breakfast Salad - 471 Calories

- ½ avocado cubed
- ¼ cucumber sliced
- ¼ cup of rocket
- ¼ cup baby spinach leaves
- 3 large radishes sliced into rounds
- 2 hard-boiled eggs, halved
- 4 tbsp fat-free chunky cottage cheese
- low-sodium salt and black pepper to taste
- 1 slice whole-wheat toast
- 1 tsp low-fat unsalted butter
- 1 tbsp balsamic vinegar

Add all the fresh ingredients to a salad bowl, toss, and drizzle with balsamic vinegar, add low-sodium salt, and black pepper to taste. Halve the hard-boiled eggs and place them on top of the salad. Spread the whole wheat toast with the teaspoon of butter and serve with the salad.

Spicy Mashed Sardines Mixed with Feta and Pickles on Whole Wheat Toast - 382 Calories

- 5 tbsp sardines, drained and mashed
- 2 slices of whole-wheat toast
- 1 tbsp feta cheese
- 2 diced pickles
- 2 tsp butter
- dash of cayenne pepper to taste and add a zing

Mash the sardines with the feta, and chopped pickles, add a touch of cayenne pepper for spice. Toast two slices of whole wheat bread and spread all with the butter. Divide the sardines and spread onto each piece of toast to enjoy.

Chocolate, Mixed Berry, Banana, Apricot, and Oats Breakfast Smoothie - 243 Calories

- 4 tbsp rolled oats
- 5 tbsp dried apricots
- 2 tbsp raspberries
- 2 tbsp blackberries
- ¼ cup chopped strawberries
- ½ small banana chopped
- 2 tsp organic honey

- ¼ unsweetened coconut water
- ¼ cup of filtered water
- 2 tsp fresh chopped mint
- 1 tsp raw organic cocoa

Blend all the ingredients until the smoothie is thick and smooth. Add to a glass and drink or pack it in a container to take with you.

Tuna, Capers, Rocket, and Feta Omelet - 482 Calories

- 3 fresh eggs
- 4 tbsp canned tuna in water without added salt
- 2 tbsp feta cheese
- 4 tbsp chopped rocket
- 2 tbsp baby spinach leaves
- 1 tsp capers
- 1 slice whole-wheat toast
- 1 tsp butter
- 1 tsp coconut oil cook with
- Black pepper to taste

Scramble the eggs in a bowl. Heat the copra oil in an omelet pan. Add the egg until it's thoroughly cooked through. Add the tuna, feta, chopped rocket, baby spinach leaves, and capers to the one half the egg mixture. Flip the free half over the ingredients to make an omelet fold. Cook on each side for 1 to 2 minutes until the omelet is cooked through.

Toast the whole wheat bread and use the butter to spread it. Cut it into triangle halves and serve it with the recent omelet.

Banana, Pomegranate Granola - 459 Calories

- 4 tbsp pomegranate seeds
- 1 large banana sliced
- 1 cup organic unsweetened granola
- 2 tsp organic honey
- 4 tbsp vanilla low-fat Greek yogurt
- 1 tbsp sunflower seeds
- 1 tbsp shredded unsweetened coconut

Place the granola in a bowl. Top with the Greek yogurt and sliced banana. Drizzle the honey over the granola and banana. Top with pomegranate seeds, sunflower seeds, and shredded coconut.

## Healthy Lunch Ideas

Lunch is an important meal because it is that the one that staves off the mid-morning hunger and gets you thru the remainder of the day. If you're getting to eat an enormous meal, this can be a far better time of the day to eat it. As you've got to urge through the subsequent half the day until supper, you'll be more likely to burn off most of the meal.

### Fasting Without Limited Calories

This way is usually done in the evening and into mid-morning the subsequent day. This fact suggests that your standard eating window would start at around 11 am. See the non-fasting healthy ideas for every day eating lunch ideas. Attempt to hamper on the calories to assist and keep your system balanced. Rather than gobbling down an excessive amount of food because you've got just come off a quick, drink a glass or two of water before eating. This fact may cause you to feel full then set about preparing your meal.

### Fasting With Limited Calories (200 to 250 Calories)

The following lunches will go down well on fasting days with limited calories as they're all 250 calories and under.

Beets, Ginger, Spring Onion With Grilled Hake - 127 Calories

- 1 grilled hake steak

- ¼ cup shredded raw beets
- 2 tbsp shredded fresh ginger root
- 3 spring onions chopped
- 1 tsp chili spice
- low-sodium salt and black pepper to taste

Preheat the grill. Prepare the hake steak with low-sodium salt, black pepper, and chili spice. Place in the grill and cook until the steak is nearly done about 10 to fifteen minutes. Turn the steak halfway through cooking to cook evenly. Top with shredded ginger root and onion. Place the dish back to the grill for an additional 5 to eight minutes. Remove from the grill, serve onto a plate, and top with fresh beets.

Golden Chocolate Avocado Smoothie - 171 Calories

- ¼ chopped avocado
- ¼ small chopped banana
- 1 cup of filtered water
- ½ cup of ice cubes
- 1 tsp turmeric
- 1 tsp raw organic cocoa
- 1 tsp vanilla extract

Add all the ingredients into the blender. Blend until the smoothie is thick and smooth. Chicken and Avocado in a Kale Wrap - 223 Calories

- ¼ avocado sliced
- ¼ cup shredded grilled chicken breast
- 2 large kale leaves
- 1 tbsp soft cottage cheese
- low-sodium salt and black pepper to taste

Mix the salt and pepper with the pot cheese. Mix the shredded chicken and avocado into the pot cheese mix. Wash and pat the kale leaves dry, then stack them on top of every other. Add the shredded chicken, avocado, and pot cheese into the center of the highest kale leaf. Fold the ruck into a wrap over the mixture and luxuriate in. You'll make three small wraps if you favor.

Chicken Liver Stuffed Zucchini Boats - 198 Calories

- 1 large zucchini
- 4 tbsp cooked chicken livers
- 2 tbsp parmesan cheese
- ¼ cup mixed salad leaves
- 1 tsp pine nuts

- ¼ cherry tomatoes halved
- 1 tbsp feta cheese
- 2 tbsp pomegranate seeds
- 3 tsp balsamic vinegar
- low-sodium salt and black pepper to taste

Preheat the grill. Halve the zucchini cutting longways into two boats. Cut out a hollow (do not go throughout the zucchini) in the middle of every ship. Put the cut-out zucchini flesh aside. Add the cooked chicken livers to the center of the zucchini, dividing them evenly between the halves. Sprinkle parmesan over the highest of the chicken livers, flavor with salt and pepper. Place the zucchini boats into the grill for 8 to 10 minutes until cooked.

While the zucchini is cooking, add the remainder of the ingredients into a salad bowl, toss, and drizzle with balsamic vinegar. Add the extra zucchini cut out from the center of the boat to the salad (chop into cubes), flavor with salt and pepper to taste. When the zucchini boats are done, serve them with the salad.

Eggplant Jalapeno and Prawn Pizza Slices— 219 Calories

- 1 large eggplant

- 2 tsp jalapeno peppers
- 6 cleaned, grilled king prawns
- 1 tbsp organic unsweetened tomato paste
- 1 tbsp shredded mozzarella cheese
- 1 tbsp parmesan cheese

Preheat the oven to 340°F. Peel the eggplant and make the slice long ways into pieces (not too thin). Spread ingredients on one side of every part. Top the component with shredded mozzarella. Chop the prawns into bits and place them on top of the element along side the jalapeno peppers. Sprinkle an honest coating of parmesan over each pizza slice. Place on a prepared baking tray and put into the oven to bake until cooked.

Healthy Lunch Ideas for Normal Eating Days (500 Calories and Under)

Tuna and Chunky Cottage Cheese Baked Potato with a Green Salad - 383 Calories

- 1 can tuna in water without salt drained
- 2 tbsp chunky fat-free plain cottage cheese
- 1 large Idaho baking potato
- ¼ cup mixed salad leaves

- ¼ cucumber diced

- ¼ green bell pepper diced

- 2 tbsp pumpkin seeds

- 2 tsp fresh basil

- 3 tsp organic balsamic vinegar

- low-sodium salt and black pepper to taste

Add salt and pepper to the pot cheese, mix in the tuna. Bake the potato and scoop out the center and blend with the tuna mixture. Add the tuna mixture to the center of the potato. Toss the salad ingredients (salad leaves, cucumber, bell pepper, pumpkin seeds, and fresh basil). Add salt and pepper to taste, drizzle with balsamic vinegar and serve with the potato.

Muscles, Lettuce, Capers, and Tomato Pita - 423 Calories

- 1 can of muscles, drained

- ¼ cup fresh shredded lettuce

- 1 whole-wheat pita

- 1 tsp capers

- ½ large tomato diced

- 4 spring onions chopped

- ¼ cucumber diced

- 4 tsp smooth cottage cheese

- 1 tsp Dijon mustard
- ¼ tsp cayenne pepper

Mix the pot cheese, Dijon mustard, and cayenne pepper. Slice the highest of the pita open and toast it until golden brown. In a bowl, toss together the muscles, lettuce, capers, tomatoes, onions, and cucumber. Mix in the mayonnaise and Dijon mustard mix. Stuff the pita pocket with muscle mixture and luxuriate in it.

Toasted Chicken and Hot English Mustard Mayo Sandwich - 464 Calories

- 2 slices of whole wheat bread
- ½ cup of shredded grilled chicken breast
- 1 tbsp low-fat mayonnaise
- 1 tsp hot English mustard
- 1 cup of oven chips
- 2 tsp unsalted butter

Cook the oven chips and spice with Cajun spice if desired. Mix the low-fat mayonnaise and hot English mustard. Add the shredded grilled chicken to the mayonnaise and mustard mix. Use the unsalted butter to butter the bread. Place the chicken on one slice of the bread, cover with the opposite piece, and grill the sandwich until it's toasted.

Tuna, Prawn, Crab, and Lobster Salad - 429 Calories

- 6 king prawns cleaned and grilled
- 4 tbsp fresh cooked crab meat
- 4 tbsp freshly cooked lobster meat
- 1 tsp capers
- 1 tsp jalapeno peppers
- 2 tsp sliced olives
- ¼ cup mixed salad leaves
- 2 tbsp feta
- ½ avocado diced
- 1 tbsp sesame seeds
- 3 tbsp low-fat mayonnaise
- 2 tsp Dijon mustard
- 1 tsp organic balsamic vinegar
- 1 tsp tomato ketchup
- 1 tsp organic honey

In a small bowl, mix the low-fat mayonnaise, Dijon mustard, ketchup, honey, and balsamic vinegar. In a salad bowl, toss together the salad ingredients, including the seafood. Drizzle with the mustard dressing and luxuriate in.

Grilled Portobello Mushrooms with Feta Cheese and Avocado Bun - 500 Calories

- 1 large portobello mushroom
- 1 tbsp feta cheese
- 1 large avocado
- 1 cup tortilla chips
- 2 tsp sliced olives
- low-sodium salt and pepper to taste

Cut the stalk from the portobello mushroom and place it on a grilling dish with the stalk side up. Add some garlic flakes, low-sodium salt, and crumble feta cheese over the mushrooms. Place it on the grill and cook it until it starts to urge soft, and therefore the feta has melted. Peel and cut the avocado in half longwise. Remove the pip, place the mushroom on the one half the avocado. Cover the mushroom with the opposite half the avocado making an avocado burger. Sever with 1 cup of tortilla chips and spice as desired.

# Healthy Dinner Ideas

Dinner should be a hearty meal, especially if you're getting to be fasting the subsequent day or through the nighttime into the subsequent day. Attempt to eat earlier in the evening to avoid getting to bed and a full stomach as this may be hard to digest and should give your problems sleeping.

## Fasting Without Limited Calories

Depending on your eating window, this may probably be your second meal of the day in a fasting period. See the non-fasting healthy ideas for standard eating day dinner ideas. Once more, attempt to control your portion sizes and gradually cut them down. Rather have a bigger lunch than a bigger dinner.

Try to eat before 7:30 pm.

## Fasting With Limited Calories (170 to 250 Calories)

The following are deliciously healthy dinner meals that offer optimum nutrition for under 250 calories. Ham and Cottage Cheese Chickpea Burger - 250 Calories

- o 1 whole wheat burger bun
- o 1 tbsp chopped cooked ham

- o 2 tsp fat-free cottage cheese
- o 1/4 cup mashed chickpeas
- o 2 lettuce leaves
- o ¼ tsp hot sauce

Drain and mash the chickpeas. Add the pot cheese, hot sauce, and ham to the chickpea mixture. Pat the chickpea mixture into a burger patty shape. Grill for 8 to 10 minutes or until the chickpea patty has heated through. Halve the burger bun, place a lettuce leaf on each half. Put the chickpea patty on rock bottom half, close the two halves and luxuriate in your burger.

Grilled Tuna on One Potato Mash - 239 Calories

- o 1 Idaho potato, boiled, and mashed
- o 1 grilled tuna steak
- o 1 cup of baby spinach leaves
- o 1 tsp pine nuts
- o 1 tbsp feta cheese
- o 1 tsp sunflower seeds
- o 1 tsp raw chopped cashew nuts
- o 2 tsp organic balsamic vinegar

Grill the tuna, seasoned with low-sodium salt and black pepper to taste. Boil and mash the Idaho potato. Toss the spinach leaves, pine nuts, sunflower seeds, cashews, and feta in a salad bowl then drizzle with balsamic vinegar. Serve the tuna on top of the mash with the tossed salad on the side.

Vegetable and 3 Cheese Tart - 215 Calories per serving

- ½ eggplant
- 3 courgettes
- ½ red bell pepper
- ½ cup baby spinach leaves
- 2 tbsp olive slices
- 1 tbsp jalapeno peppers
- 1 roll of puff pastry
- 4 tbsp feta cheese
- 4 tbsp fat-free cottage cheese
- 2 tbsp parmesan cheese This makes three servings.

Preheat the oven to 300°F. Prepare a baking tray with cooking spray. Roll out the filo pastry and place it in pie shape at rock bottom of the baking tray. Place the pastry into the oven until it starts to urge brown. Cook the vegetables in a skillet with copra oil over medium heat and when cooked, mix in the cheese, and place them in the pie shell. Mix in olive slices and crumble feta over the vegetable mix. Then sprinkle it with parmesan cheese and place the pie back in the oven and cook for 8-10 minutes until the cheese has melted. Remove from the oven and serve.

Asparagus, Green Bean, and Poached Egg Salad - 218 Calories

- 5 fresh grilled asparagus spears
- 1 cup grilled green beans
- 2 poached egg
- ½ cup baby spinach leaves
- ¼ cup rocket
- 4 tsp Dijon mustard

Lay a bed of baby spinach leaves mixed with rocket leaves. Place the grilled asparagus and beans onto the mixed rucks. Place the warm poached egg on the top, drizzle with Dijon mustard and enjoy. Grilled Turkey Breast with Boiled Garlic and Ginger Butter Baby Potatoes - 250 Calories

- 4 washed and boiled baby potatoes
- ½ grilled turkey breast cut into slices
- 1 tsp grated fresh ginger root
- 1 tsp organic crushed garlic
- 3 tsp unsalted butter
- low-sodium salt and black pepper to taste

Place the recent grilled and sliced turkey breast on a plate with the boiled baby potatoes. In a pot, melt the butter with the grated ginger root and garlic. When the butter is cooked, pour the mixture over the baby potatoes and serve. You'll add some mixed salad leaves if you would like.

Dinner Ideas for Normal Eating Days (500 Calories and Under)

The following dinner ideas are quick and straightforward to make, are under 500 calories and high in healthy nutrition.

Bison Burger with Cajun Oven Baked Potato Wedges and Sour Cream - 500 Calories

- 1 bison burger patty
- 1 whole-wheat bun
- 1 tbsp Dijon mustard
- 1 large pickle, thinly sliced
- 1 large washed lettuce leaf
- 1 slice of a large tomato
- 1 cup of oven-baked potato wedges
- 1 tsp Cajun spice
- 3 tbsp low-fat sour cream
- 1 tsp finely chopped fresh dill

Halve the burger bun and spread each half with Dijon mustard. Grill the bison burger patty and before stacking it on the rock bottom of the halved burger bun. Top the cake with a lettuce leaf, tomato slice, sliced pickle. In a bowl, mix the soured cream and dill. Bake the potato wedges consistent with the pack, spice with Cajun spice, and drizzle with the soured cream and fresh chive sauce.

Surf and Turf with a Baked Potato and Sour Cream - 500 Calories

- 1 prime cut steak - grilled and spiced to your liking
- 1 large baking potato, baked until soft
- 6 large grilled prawns
- 1 tsp garlic butter
- 1 tsp unsalted butter
- 1 tbsp sour cream
- 1 cup cooked green beans

Cook the steak and baking potato to your liking. Grill the prawns and warmth the spread when the prawns are nearly cooked. Cook the green beans to your liking and serve them onto a plate. Add the steak, prawns, and baked potatoes. Pour the heated spread over the prawns. Add unsalted butter, soured cream, salt, and pepper to the potato and serve while nice and hot.

Quick Black Bean Chili - 343 Calories

- ¼ cup of cooked brown rice
- ½ white onion chopped
- 2 large fresh tomatoes chopped
- 1 can black beans
- 2 tsp crushed garlic
- 1 tbsp of chili powder (strength to your taste)
- 2 tbsp of organic honey
- 2 tbsp jalapeno peppers
- 2 tbsp organic balsamic vinegar
- 2 tsp paprika
- 2 tbsp sour cream
- 4 tbsp of feta
- ½ thinly sliced avocado
- 8 sprigs of fresh mint
- ¼ cup of warm water

This recipe makes 4 servings.

Cook the rice when the chili has fifteen minutes of cooking time left. In a large pot, bring the nice and cozy water to boil, add the onion, black beans, crushed garlic, flavored, honey, balsamic vinegar, and paprika. Allow the chili to cook for 1-hour half-hour or until the beans are soft. Serve with a dollop of soured cream, crumbled feta, avocado, and a few fresh mints.

Avocado, Bacon, Rocket, and Feta Tortilla Pizza - 342 Calories

- 1 whole wheat tortilla
- ¼ avocado thinly sliced
- ¼ cup crisped bacon pieces
- 4 tbsp rocket
- 2 tbsp feta
- 4 tbsp shredded mozzarella
- 2 tsp organic tomato paste
- low-sodium salt and black pepper to taste

Preheat the oven to 340°F. Spread the tortilla with the ingredient, top with mozzarella, avocado, bacon, rocket, and crumble the feta cheese over the highest. Place it in the oven and cook until all the ingredients are cooked, and therefore the tortilla is golden brown.

Spicy Mince Meat Pancakes - 370 Calories

- Make a pancake mixture (2 eggs, ¼ cup flour, ¼ cup reduced-fat milk)
- 1 cup mince
- 5 basil leaves
- 1 tsp dried oregano
- 1 tsp chili powder
- 1 tsp jalapeno peppers
- 1 tsp capers
- ¼ cup mixed salad leaves
- ¼ cucumber chopped
- 1 celery stalk chopped
- 1 tsp balsamic vinegar

Make two pancakes. Then cook the mince with the herbs and spices. Dish the mince out evenly into the center of every pancake. Add jalapeno peppers and capers to every pancake and serve. Toss the salad greens together (salad leaves, cucumber, and celery) then drizzle balsamic vinegar over them. Serve the pancakes with the tossed salad on the side.

## Healthy Smoothies

These smoothies are often wont to replace breakfast or lunch. They will even be used as a snack.

Smoothies are fun to make, and you'll experiment with different fruit, nut, and vegetable blends. Add differing types of nut milk, nut creams, yogurt, and so on. They're always tastier once you add seeds.

Keep the ingredients healthy and in snack or meal calorie requirements. They're an excellent thanks to getting all of your nutrition requirements specific the day. They will even be taken as an on the go meal or snack.

Smoothies may only be drunk in regular eating periods or windows. As they're a snack that contains carbs, they can't be drunk in the fasting periods.

They are easy to make as you set all the ingredients into a blender, then blend until smooth and thick. Leftover smoothie mixture is often kept in an airtight container in the refrigerator for up to 2 days.

Smoothies with added protein powder are excellent thanks to aiding muscle recovery after a troublesome workout, long run, bike ride, etc. they will also offer you that added boost of energy if you're feeling tired and run down. Smoothie Ingredients

Smoothies can contain any fruit, berry, nut, seed, protein, whey powder, yogurt, etc.

Fruit and berries are often either frozen or fresh. Avoid canned fruit or berries and make sure the products don't have any added sugar, flavors, or colorants.

Here are a couple of samples of the main popular smoothie ingredients:

- Berries
- Raspberries
- Blackberries
- Blueberries
- Strawberries Fruit
- Banana (they are great for thickening and sweetening a smoothie)
- Avocado
- Pear
- Plum
- Peach
- Apple
- Pineapple
- Melon (yellow)

- Papaya
- Watermelon
- Grapes
- Pomegranate seeds
- Kiwi
- Mango
- Coconut
- Nuts
- Cashews
- Macadamia
- Walnuts
- Almonds
- Pecan
- Pistachios
- Brazil nuts
- Seeds
- Chia
- Sunflower
- Pinenut
- Pumpkin
- Sesame
- Fennel

- Vegetables
- Kale
- Spinach
- Cabbage  Broccoli
- Tomato
- Celery
- Carrot
- Raddish
- Horseradish
- Cucumber
- Spring onion
- Artichoke
- Garlic
- Rocket  Capers
- Herbs
- Mint
- Basil
- Oregano
- Parsley
- Ginger
- Rosemary
- Cardamom

- Mustard seeds
- Chives
- Spices
- Turmeric
- Paprika
- Cayenne pepper
- Ground cinnamon
- Allspice
- Chili powder
- Chili seeds
- Ground ginger
- Garlic powder
- Cumin
- Dill
- Low sodium salt
- Black pepper
- White pepper
- Worcestershire sauce
- Soy sauce
- Tomato ketchup
- Mustard
- Liquids

- Filtered water
- Ice cubes
- Almond milk
- Hemp milk
- Rice milk
- Oat milk
- Coconut milk
- Coconut cream
- Coconut water
- Low-fat milk
- Cream
- Fruit juice
- Vegetable juice
- Other
- Vanilla essence
- Pure vanilla
- Organic Balsamic vinegar
- Curry powder
- Vegetable oil
- Protein whey powder (all flavors)
- Plain low-fat Greek yogurt
- Low-fat cheese

- Fat-free pot cheese
- Flavored low-fat yogurt
- Sugar-free frozen dessert (all flavors)
- Raw organic chocolate
- Dark chocolate chips
- Dark chocolate blocks
- Organic honey
- Desiccated coconut
- Coconut flakes
- Fresh chilis
- Smoothie Ideas

These are tasty smoothies that are filled with good nutrition, taste great, and 350 calories or under.

Avocado, Banana, Chocolate, and Ginger Smoothie - 312 Calories

- ½ banana
- ½ avocado
- 1 tbsp grated fresh ginger root
- 1 tsp sunflower seeds
- 1 tsp chia seeds
- 1 tsp vanilla extract

- ¼ cup unsweetened almond milk
- ¼ cup of filtered water

## Peach, Blueberry Cheesecake Smoothie - 350 Calories

- ½ banana
- 1 peach
- ½ cup blueberries
- 1 tbsp sesame seeds
- 1 tbsp organic honey
- ½ cup low-fat milk
- ¼ cup of ice cubes
- ¼ cup sugar-free vanilla ice cream

## The Green and Gold Smoothie - 124 Calories

- ½ banana
- ¼ cup kale
- ¼ cup baby spinach leaves
- ¼ cucumber
- ½ green bell pepper
- 1 tsp fresh dill
- 2 tsp turmeric
- ½ cup of filtered water
- ¼ cup unsweetened coconut water

- low-sodium salt and black pepper to taste

Berry, Nut, and Seed Coconut Cream Smoothie with a Zing - 319 Calories

- ¼ cup blackberries
- ¼ cup blueberries
- ¼ cup raspberries
- ¼ cup pomegranate seeds
- 1 tsp sunflower seeds
- 1 tsp fennel seeds
- 1 tsp sesame seeds
- 3 tsp raw cashew nuts
- 2 tsp pecan nuts
- 2 tbsp unsweetened shredded coconut
- 4 tbsp unsweetened coconut cream
- ¼ cup unsweetened almond milk
- ¼ cup of filtered water
- 3 tsp organic honey
- dash of cayenne pepper

Tomato Beet Vegetable Cocktail Smoothie - 154 Calories

- 1 carrot
- 2 celery stalks

- 2 medium tomatoes
- ¼ cup baby spinach leaves
- ½ green bell pepper
- ¼ cucumber
- ¼ cup grated fresh beets
- 3 tsp fresh basil
- ½ cup of filtered water
- ¼ cup fresh orange juice
- low-sodium salt and ground black pepper to taste

Tropical Coconut Cream and Ginger Smoothie - 350 Calories

- ½ cup of pineapple
- ½ banana
- ½ mango
- 1 kiwifruit
- ¼ papaya
- 1 tbsp unsweetened shredded coconut
- 1 tbsp grated ginger root
- 1 tsp ground cinnamon
- 2 tsp organic honey
- ¼ cup fresh orange juice
- ¼ cup fresh lime juice

# Beverages In Fasting Periods

There are some beverages you'll drink in fasting periods, and a few you want to avoid. There are substances not be added to any beverages in fast and others which can be added. Here are some ideas on what you ought to and will not be drinking in fasting periods.

- Water
- Water should be drunk continuously in the day, even once you aren't fasting.
- Water is usually best drunk as natural, filtered, or spring water, which will be either carbonated or still.
- You May Add
- Lemon
- Lime
- Cucumber slices
- The water is often carbonated

You May Not Add

- Artificial sweeteners
- Colorants
- Artificial flavors
- Fruit

- Berries
- Tea

There are a couple of teas that ought to be avoided and people who will be consumed. It's best to drink the tea black with a touch of cold water if it must be cooled down. Oolong tea

- Black tea
- Normal tea
- Green tea
- Cinnamon tea
- Peppermint tea
- Spearmint tea

You May Add

- Stevia
- Cinnamon
- Nutmeg
- Lemon juice

You May Not Add

- Artificial sweeteners
- Milk
- Cream

- Artificial flavors
- Fruit
- Herbs
- Spices
- Coffee

Black coffee helps to stay you alert and awake. It can also aid in weight loss.

You May Add

- Stevia
- Cinnamon
- Nutmeg
- Lemon juice

You May Not Add

- Artificial sweeteners
- Milk
- Cream
- Artificial flavors
- Herbs
- Spices

# Concerns In Fasting

One of the leading causes of individuals abandoning fasting is because they get headaches, feel nauseous, or cannot debar hunger.

Here are a couple of tips to assist and get you thru a couple of concerns.

## Constipation

Constipation does happen in fasting, especially once you first start.

Try these tips:

- Increase your fiber content in your eating windows.
- Drink soda water.
- Use fennel seeds together with your smoothies or sprinkle them over your food.
- Drink hot coffee.
- Drink black or tea.

## Dizziness

You may feel a touch dizzy or such as you have vertigo in the fasting periods. You'll even feel light-headed whenever you get up or get a blood rush to the top. This effect is often usually caused by dehydration.

Try these tips:

- Increase your fluid intake.
- Drink mint in your water in the eating windows.
- Take liver salts in the eating window.
- Cut down on coffee and tea intake for a short time.

**Fatigue or Lethargy**

You will feel a touch tired or lethargic in fasting periods. You'll even be lacking some vital nutrients. Increase your nutrient intake in non-fasting periods.

Try these tips:

- Increase your fluid intake.
- Eat high energy foods in your eating window, and a minimum of an hour before your fasting period is close to starting.
- Splash cold water on your face.
- Do some light exercise.
- Take supplements in your eating window.

## Headaches

Headaches are another common occurrence in fasting. Your body goes through a period of withdrawal and isn't won't to being starved of food.

Try these tips:

- Drink more water.
- Drink drinking water in your non-fasting periods.

## Muscle Cramps or Spasms

Fasting also means lowering salt and a few minerals. This fact will cause muscle cramps and muscle spasms.

Try these tips:

- Take Epsom salts twice every week in your eating windows.
- Increase your magnesium intake in your eating windows.

## Nausea

You may experience nausea if hunger sets in; otherwise, you may experience migraine symptoms.

Try these tips:

- Drink peppermint tea.
- Drink liver salts in your eating window.

**Hunger**

The most common concern or complaint is feeling hungry. There are tons you'll do to prevent you from feeling hungry and alleviate the hunger pangs.

Try these tips:

- Increase your fiber content in your eating windows.
- Eat more slow-release carbs a minimum of an hour before the fasting period begins.
- Drink soda water.
- Drink tea.
- Drink coffee.
- Add cinnamon to your coffee or tea.
- Distract yourself by keeping busy with a hobby.
- Get some light exercise in or choose an extended walk.
- Meditate.
- Visit a lover.

## Sleeping Problems

If you're fasting in the night, you'd have probably started fasting around 7:30 pm. Move that period up to a minimum of 9 pm and have a light-weight snack and a cup of chamomile tea before bed.

Read a book and switch off all electronics, which will be disturbing your sleeping pattern. Confirm your room is cold, even in winter, your place must be fresh to take care of a top-quality sleep pattern.

Keep a fresh bottle of water next to your bed just if you get thirsty in the night, so you are doing not need to rise and pour one.

Learn sleep meditation to relax your body and assist you in falling asleep to sleep.

# Dealing with Unpleasant Side Effects

Earlier in the introduction, I promised you unbiased information on intermittent fasting. Keep thereupon promise; this chapter will delve into the possible adverse side effects of fasting intermittently. Some people that swear by this practice might not be willing to admit that there are unpleasant side effects of fasting intermittently. But that might be myopic and withholding vital information.

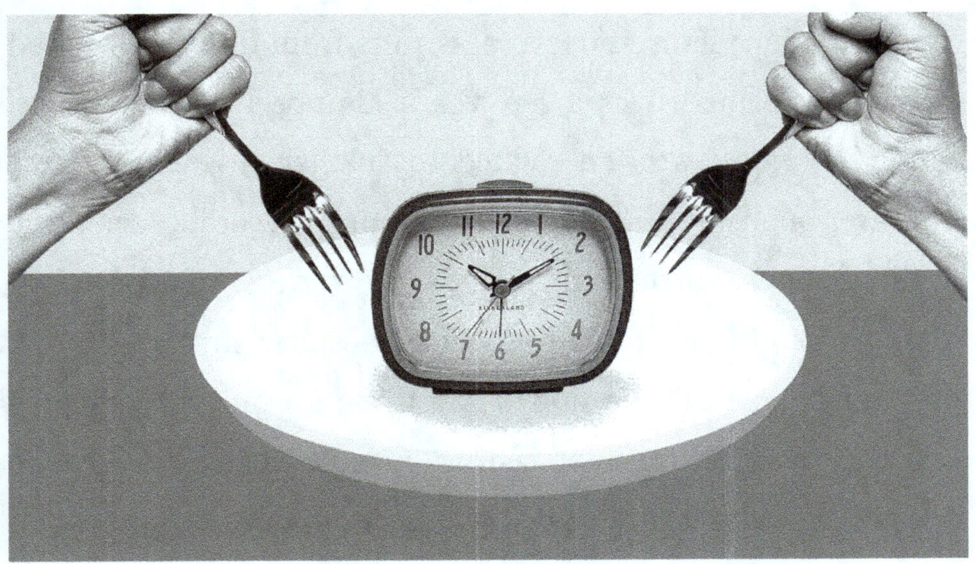

It's essential to means that the overall downsides of intermittent fasting are common to all or any women no matter age. While women of child-bearing age may need effects on their reproductive hormones, post-menopausal women or older women might not get to worry about reproduction. However, they experience frequent changes in their moods, difficulty in sleeping, and occasional headaches.

After a comprehensive review of several scientific studies on women's health, fasting, and aging, researchers weren't ready to find any significant adverse effect of intermittent fasting and point to a scarcity of research on the subject (Journal of Mid-Life Health, 2016). These sorts of scientific reviews are beneficial for getting the unbiased information that provides you a broader picture of several results from different related studies performed over a few years. Comprehensive reviews hamper prejudices often related to smaller researchers that will are sponsored by interest groups. Overall, scientific studies show encouraging leads to different aspects of women's health, including psychological state, physical fitness, and weight loss. That's not to say there are not any adverse side effects of intermittent fasting. It only means the adverse side effects of intermittent fasting are common to women of all ages – both pre and post-menopausal women and depend mainly on the individual woman.

With that being said, not everyone who practices intermittent fasting will have a negative side effect. These differ from person to person. The important thing is being conscious of these adverse side effects and learning the way to handle them if they occur. Also, remember that the majority of the off-putting impacts of intermittent fast don't last beyond the primary few days. Every week or two, your body would have adjusted to your new eating schedule, and any adverse effects will gradually subside until things feel back to normal. So, it's crucial to permit your body a while to regulate rather than trying intermittent fasting for one or two days and throwing in the towel.

Here is the way to affect a number of the common negative side effects you'll likely encounter as you begin your new eating habits.

## Hunger

One of the primary not-so-fun and most blatant results of fasting is hunger. This side effect is difficult because going without food longer than your body is conditioned to will end in an uncomfortable desire for love or money to eat. All of your life, you've got programmed your body to expect food at certain times throughout the day. It might be weird if you suddenly change your eating pattern, and your body accepts the change without putting up a minimum of a touch resistance. If your body doesn't get food at the time it usually does, a hormone called ghrelin – the hunger hormone – will start acting up to remind you that you simply should supply your body with food. This "acting up" or reminder to erode your usual time will continue until your brain convinces ghrelin to accept your new eating schedule simply. But until then, you'll likely feel intense hunger but don't worry; it'll pass. You'll get to tap into your reserve of mental strength to remain committed to your course.

To effectively handle hunger pangs, drink more water, or any qualifying beverage on intermittent fasting. Doing so will help to suppress hunger pangs. Very often, the sensation of hunger isn't necessarily a sign that you simply are hungry; it'd be a small dip in your blood glucose level – something that water or other non-calorie liquids can look out of.

To help delay hunger on your fasting days or in the fasting window (depending on the sort of fasting regimen you select to follow), make sure that you include adequate amounts of healthy fats, carbs, and proteins in your meals before commencing your fast. Also, when fasting, try to take your mind off food. Combining low-impact exercises with fasting can assist in giving you the boost you would like to travel through your day without feeling too uncomfortable. Getting enough sleep also will help you throughout the day; there's nothing that will upset your day entirely lack of sleep in the dark and having to fast. That's an open invitation for fatigue and hunger!

## Frequent Urination

As with hunger, it's also expected to experience a rise in the number of times you urinate. There's no mystery here as intermittent fasting takes that you simply increase your intake of water and other liquids to remain hydrated. This effect may successively increase the frequency of urination. Keep drinking your water, and don't avoid bathroom visits. Holding it for too long can weaken your bladder muscles, and trying not to drink water will soon cause you to be dehydrated and supply subsequent side effects – both bad!

## Headaches

Intermittent fasting can make your blood glucose to take a nosedive. This fact introduces stress on your body, your brain will release stress hormones, and you'll likely experience a point of headache. Dehydration can cause headaches in intermittent fasting as your body tells you it lacks adequate water.

To reduce the occurrence of headaches, attempt to minimize stress on your body. It's okay to exercise in fasting, but excessive exercise can trigger an excessive amount of stress. Also, attempt to keep your body hydrated in the least times by drinking enough water. But don't chug water in a rush and don't drink water excessively. An excessive amount of water may result in an imbalance in your mineral and body water ratio.

## Cravings

It is normal to experience quite usual cravings for food in your fasting window. This fact is often a biological and psychological response to the sensation of deprivation that's often related to going without food. And since your body is all bent get glucose, you would possibly notice that you simply crave for more sugar or carbohydrates. These cravings don't mean that you simply are less committed to your goals. Instead, cravings happen to remind you that you simply are human. Even ardent practitioners of intermittent fasting experience cravings from time to time.

When you start looking for something, remind yourself of your goal and distract yourself from food-related topics. Keep your mind engrossed with other non-food related activities like hobbies, talking an enter nature, or getting to sleep for a short time. In your eating window, you'll treat yourself to a healthy bite of what you crave to attenuate the intensity of the craving or longing. Remind yourself in your fasting window that you simply will soon eat what you long for, so there's no need dwelling thereon or giving it an excessive amount of thought when it's not yet time to eat. Remind your body that you simply are not any longer an adolescent or a young adult. You've got had many experiences in curbing your cravings, and this case isn't an exception.

## Heartburn, Bloating, and Constipation

Occasionally, heartburn can occur when your stomach produces acids for digestion of your food, but there's no food present in the stomach to be digested. Bloating and constipation usually go hand in hand and may also occur in some cases. Together, these two can cause you to feel very uncomfortable.

Drinking adequate amounts of water can reduce the danger of heartburn, bloating, and constipation. Heartburns also can be minimized by lowering on spicy foods in your eating window. If you experience heartburn in intermittent fasting, here's something you'll try before getting to sleep. Prop yourself up once you lie to sleep. But don't use pillows to prop yourself as which will put more pressure on your stomach and increase the discomfort. Use a specially designed wedge or use a 6-inch block or something almost like elevate your head as you lie. Doing this may make gravity minimize the backward flow of your stomach contents into your gullet. Propping yourself in this manner should bring you relief from heartburn. However, if heartburn, bloating, and constipation persist, consult your doctor immediately.

## Binging

Eating an excessive amount as soon because the fasting window is over is typically related to first-timers to fasting. The extreme hunger of fasting can drive you to dine in a rush when breaking, and you'll find yourself overeating. In some cases, binging is often a result of an easy misunderstanding of the fundamentals of intermittent fasting. They assume that they will eat the maximum amount as they need in the eating window since the no-eating window will look out of calories. This misunderstanding can deprive you of gaining any significant benefits that accompany fasting intermittently, especially if you're looking to shed some weight. Binging or overeating in your eating window will reverse all the diligence you set in in the fast.

To avoid binging, make sure that the dimensions and meals are planned well before the eating window. Don't start fasting without knowing what portion you're getting to consume at the top. Waiting until you'll eat to make a decision about what to eat and the way much to eat can cause overeating because your food choices are going to be primarily influenced by how hungry you are feeling.

## Low Energy

Feeling exhausted may be a standard a part of fasting. Until your body gets won't to sourcing its fuel from fat storage, you're likely to experience some decline in your energy levels. Usually, they revisit up in a few days.

To help stay energized, tailor your activities to remain low-key, a minimum of initially. There's no got to push yourself to prove that you simply are a robust woman. Deciding to practice intermittent fasting is enough proof that you simply are mentally, emotionally, and physically healthy. Since you're not in competition with anyone, it's in your best interest to conserve energy the maximum amount as possible. Get a massage, spend time relaxing in bed, or sleeping in if you've got to. These little activities can go an extended way to keep you energized.

## Feeling Cold

Some people experience an additional feeling of cold in fasting. If you experience this, there's no cause for alarm. It'd be a result of the drop by your blood glucose level. Usually, blood flow to your internal fat storage is increased in fasting. This increase results in fat moved to parts of the body where it needs to be used as energy. This effect will make other parts of your body that have less fat storage to experience cold. So, if you feel cold in your fingers or toes, it's your body doing its fat burning process for your good.

To help reduce the cold, place on layers, stay in warm areas, drink hot coffee or tea (with no calories), or take a hot shower. It's important to keep in mind that feeling cold is simply a result of intermittent fasting and doesn't mean you're ill. So, avoid the urge to self-medicate. If the cold feeling persists even in your non-fasting days or in your eating window, consult your doctor.

## Mood Swing

Imagine the following combinations of stress on your body caused by the dip in your blood glucose. Your hormones are going berserk from the varied reactions happening in your body as a result of not eating normally or on schedule. And the lethargic feeling from lack of food, hunger, and cravings that are always telling you to eat. Not having the ability to socialize with others freely due to your new eating pattern, you can't wine and dine at social events if it's outside your eating window! All of those can cause a mental state of feeling annoyed or irritated.

The surest thanks to minimizing mood swings resulting from intermittent fasting are to deliberately keep your attention off issues that set you jittery and specialize in what you're doing and what causes you to be happy. The more you retain your mind bound up in gratitude and appreciation, the higher you'll feel. So, in your fasting window, be deliberate about engaging in things that lift your spirits and keep your mind on happy and productive thoughts.

## Bottom Line

Intermittent fasting may be a lifestyle regimen that's safe for older practitioners. It's a medical intervention that will cause improvements in many aspects of a woman's health. However, it's not suitable for each person. If you notice that you simply have severe adverse reactions to intermittent fasting, it's in your best interest to desist directly and consult your doctor. No rule makes it compulsory to finish a quick once you start. You'll break in the middle of your fasting window (even if it's just that day) if you'll not endure unpleasant side effects and check out again at a later time.

While it's okay to offer your body a couple of weeks to urge won't to your new eating pattern, it's also crucial to pay close attention to what your body is telling you. Thankfully, as an older woman with experience, you'll tell when something works for you. You recognize once you can plan to something, and once you can't find the motivation to follow through. I think that, as a lady with an incredible wealth of experience, you'll find the strength to stay to your resolve reasonably.

# Changing Your Habits and Achieving Your Goals

The best way to get rid of old habits is to change your mindset.

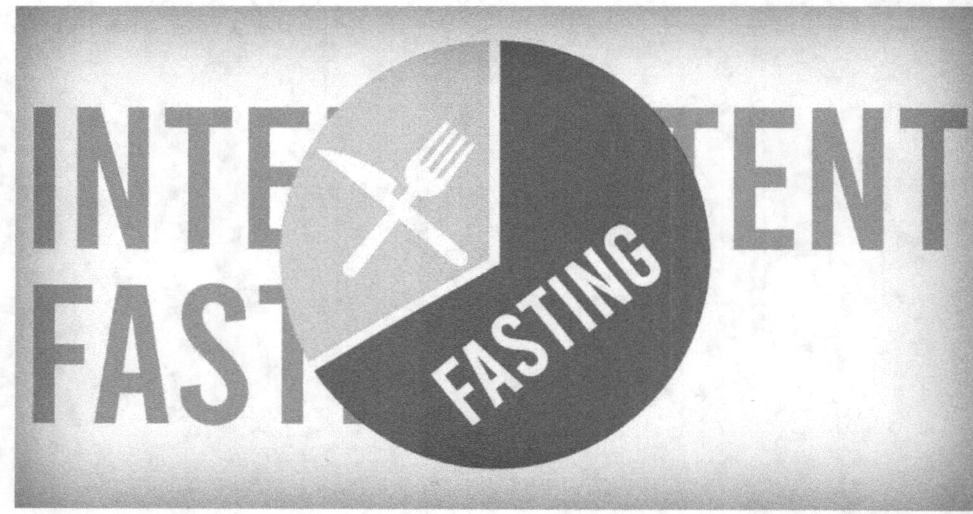


## Take Control of Your Habits

Bad habits get ingrained into your subconscious as they're repeated day in and outing. Bite your nails, sucking your thumb, eating three large meals each day, and so on. Recurring patterns create habits throughout your time. These habits are started by our parents growing up, my nerves, anxiety, or a way of support. Breaking them doesn't happen in a day and can take time. Some habits you're doing not even know you are doing as they need become a reflex. This way includes the way you eat, cook, and even shop.

Habits, regardless of what they're, are often broken. You only got to want to interrupt the routine, have the strength to break the pattern, and believe that you simply can.

# Breaking Bad Habits

Instead of trying to interrupt them, replace them with healthier ones.

Here are some recommendations on the way to take hold of your habits to vary them.

### The Triggers

Become conscious of your triggers. Once you're aware of why you are doing what you are doing, you'll find how around them. Habits are an individual's little comfort devices and intrinsically are very easy to fall back to. To vary them, we'd like to develop new comforts, and at midlife, it becomes quite a challenge to do.

One way to retrain the response to a trigger would be to possess a countermeasure in situ. For instance, if you discover yourself reaching for dessert after supper, stop, and ask yourself why you have the dessert. Are you continue to hungry? If so, get something with less sugar and calories in, or reach for fruit instead.

If you want something sweet, have a glass of infused water and believe what healthy snacks you'll eat instead. Grapes are a healthier alternative to sweets, chocolates, or carbonated drinks.

Don't think, "I must eat something healthy." Instead, think, "I would much prefer something healthy to eat."

When you shopping, don't think, "I must like better to take this product." Reach for the healthier alternative and think, "Ah! This way is often my new favorite brand."

## Dealing with Triggers

Most people are conscious of their triggers on some level. The simplest solution would be to avoid situations that trigger bad habits. The thing is, in the real world, you're always getting to encounter a trigger or two somewhere. It's like trying to avoid an individual you are doing not like, unless you're getting to change continents, even then that's no guarantee.

If you can't avoid them, find out how to affect them. As per the section above, have a coping mechanism, you'll fall back on aside from the bad habit. If you discover you're unable to resist hotdogs, once you pass a hotdog vendor, carry a nutritious snack with you. A couple of squares of bittersweet chocolate could do the trick or a couple of berries or nuts. Take it out and eat it as you travel by or dial a lover to occupy your mind while walking past.

Find a mantra that most accurately fits you and talk yourself through it once you end up in a situation that triggers a habit. You're trying to combat the signs of aging, not just on the surface but on the in. To do that, you simply need to break bad eating habits, including the way you cook, the groceries you purchase, and eating out habits. Most decent restaurants and even fast-food places try to supply healthy menu choices. Consider trying something new on the menu for a replacement and improved you!

## Switching the Bad for the Good

In theory, it sounds relatively easy to do, but actually, it's tough. You've got spent most of your life eating the way you are doing, shopping the way you are doing, and so on. By now, your life works on autopilot as you undergo your habitual daily routine. Now you're trying to slowly change your entire lifestyle and undo all those years of mental wiring.

It is getting to take strength, commitment, and perseverance. But the top results of intermittent fasting and choosing a healthier lifestyle do justify the means. One of the simplest ways to start is to consider it as switching out this product for a replacement product, quite like switching out your laundry detergents to undertake a replacement brand. Don't believe it as breaking bad habits or a diet. Instead, consider your new lifestyle as trying something new.

## Change Your Mindset

You have had a particular mindset for years, and now you're changing it, retraining your brain, setting new routines, and developing new comfort zones. The human psyche is complex, and humans are their own worst enemies. Believe it or not, you're getting to come up against resistance to all or any of your changes. Even the littlest of changes may have some sort of resistance. The most challenging part is it's not resistance from a moody teenager or partner. And the opposition to vary will come from in you!

You can start to vary your mindset by trying several following methods:

## Have a Transparent Vision

One thing on your side, once you reach midlife, is that your taste changes. Usually, at midlife, an individual starts to seek out those foods that when agreed with them not do. While other foods may become more appealing, your tastes can change, and food might not taste an equivalent. Now's the shortest time to embrace new eating habits. You've got the right excuse to use against your inner rebel.

If eating meat has begun to cause indigestion, try substituting it with a plant-based alternative. Chickpeas make an excellent, tasty, meat alternative. If you're keen on bacon, you don't need to provides it up entirely; once more, try a plant alternative, like eggplant. Find the foods that best suit you and your new tastes, don't be afraid to undertake something new. This fact is often a replacement phase of your life cycle. Not only are you turning over a replacement leaf, but you're going to know this new you.

Parents will have skilled the various phases in their kid's life, and as they grew, you had to grow with them. You adapted and evolved around the different stages. This fact is often tons like that, only now you've reached a replacement phase of your life. And to enjoy your life with optimum health, changes are essential. Even people who have led a comparatively healthy lifestyle, trained a day, and conquered mountains, will need to adapt at now in their life.

Your body is changing from inside, and what worked for you before menopause will presumably not work for you now. You can't let it defeat you or get you down; you would like to embrace it and set your vision on where you go from here. Make an inventory of the significant changes you feel you would like to deal with. Include what you'd wish to change and note any health issues you simply think you would like to deal with.

## Midlife Vision Board

Vision boards are tons of fun and are trending lately. They provide you something to aspire to, and as you notice changes in your lifestyle change, it is an excellent visualization tool. There's nothing more motivating than actually seeing the changes and the way much you've got transformed from point A to where you currently are.

# Chart Your Progress

Set a date for once every week, bi-weekly, or monthly where you're taking note of your changes. Weigh yourself, measure yourself, note further you'll walk more now, and so on. Document how you are feeling. Are you sleeping better? Does one desire you've got more energy now?

List all the changes you made for the period, how you adapted to them, and any new changes or modifications you would like.

Make sure to write down the days you slipped up, anything you had a tough time with, and, therefore, the things that just didn't meet your needs. It will appear to be diligent, but you'll be amazed how encouraging it's once you lay it all out. It also gives you a baseline from which to figure from and how to make adjustments.

# Set Obtainable Goals

One of the worst belongings you can do is about your targets or goals too high. Keep a transparent vision in mind of what your overall mark is. Then set weekly or instead monthly targets to strive for.

Make weekly goals about small adjustments to your lifestyle, like changing dairy products for nut milk. Make your monthly targets about losing weight or rather centimeters and your fitness levels.

Breaking down your lifestyle goals into smaller obtainable, and doable chunks make achieving your overall goal more realistic. Having small goals is analogous to breaking down a project into milestones. You recognize where the project goes and, therefore, how it should find yourself and the steps to take to urge there.

Having smaller goals helps continue your morale because there's nothing like achieving that first milestone. That's once you know you're on the right path, and it causes you to want to urge to the subsequent milestone.

It also keeps you in a positive can-do mindset as once you've reached subsequent few, you're well on your thanks to the ultimate goal post.

## A New Daily Routine

When you change your eating habits, it affects your daily routine, especially when intermittent fasting. You've got to schedule your meals around your fasting days also as your social calendar. If you're unsure if you'll be ready to resist temptation, it's best to schedule family outings, lunches, and get-togethers on non-fasting days. There are getting to be times once you cannot do that. Instead, attempt to be flexible regarding your scheduled fasting days.

### Your Daily To-*Do* List

You need to arrange your schedule to start a replacement routine. The primary thing you ought to do is create your daily task list. This fact is often everything you are doing throughout the day and which days you are doing what tasks on.

While fasting shouldn't interfere together with your daily routine, it could interfere together with your social one. To profit from intermittent fasting, you would like to make it fit into your life. To settle on or modify an idea to fit your needs best, you would like to determine what your current routine is so you'll adapt it to suit your new lifestyle.

While jotting down what all you are doing in the day every day, here are some inquiries to confine mind:

- How does the morning start? Write down the overall time you rise. Any pre-breakfast tasks?
- Do you create breakfast every morning?

- Do you've got kids you would like to urge off to high school, college, or work?
- Do you've got a partner that must get off to work?
- If you're working, what's your morning routine to urge ready?
- Do you've got any work function commitments in the next one to 3 months?
- Do you've got any social or family functions/gatherings/commitments in the subsequent three months?
- When are grocery days?  When are the laundry days?
- What housework does one do, and when?
- Do you exercise? If so, how frequently?
- What hobbies does one have?
- Do you've got club membership, and are there any club engagements coming up?
- List any events you'll have arising, holidays, sports tournaments, sport commitments, etc.

Include everything that you simply might imagine has relevance to your schedule that you know you are doing like clockwork. Events like weddings, engagement parties, birthday functions, work functions all got to be jotted down.

As do any social engagements, book clubs, girls' nights out, etc. all of them play an important part in having a well-adjusted fasting schedule that works well with and for you.

## Create a Replacement Schedule

Choose the sort of fasting plan you think that you'll be ready to start with and stick with. Before you plan to time windows for fasting and eating, assess your current schedule. You'll get to adjust your schedule and perhaps even modify your fasting decide to find a compromise for your program.

Before you begin making up your schedule, it's time to take stock of you. Take notes of the days for the day you are feeling you've got the very best energy levels. This way is often the time of day to do the work, like exercises and training your mind to interrupt old habits to make room for brand spanking new ones. Use your afternoons to line up menus for the subsequent day, make appointments, watch the kid's sports games, or meet with friends for tea.

Do things that don't take tons of energy, but that also keeps you active and your mind working.

You should include a variety of things on your schedule like:

- The time you would like to awaken each morning so you'll set your alarm.
- Any appointments you, your partner, or kids may have every day.
- Shopping for groceries, or any household, school, or office supplies you'll need.
- Family commitments for the day or evening
- Upcoming events you would like to urge yourself and your family ready for.
- New foods you'd wish to try every day
- Any changes you'd wish to make on certain days which will ease you into your new healthy lifestyle
- Exercise for the day.

Set a time window for bedtimes. This way might seem a touch infantile, but you would like to start out getting a simple sleep pattern going. If you create a concerted effort to urge to bed at a daily time each night, your body will soon adapt to the present routine. You'll end up beginning to feel tired by a particular point of the evening.

## It Is All Up to You

Reading self-help books, laying out the groundwork, and setting goals is the easy part. The hard part is putting it all into practice, which is all up to you. Now that you simply have chosen your fasting plan, decided upon a diet, and set your new routine, it's time to take the subsequent step.

It is time to urge real and set a reasonable start date. Attend bed the night before and believe sleep as your cocoon. Subsequent morning you're getting to awaken, taking over the primary day of your new lifestyle. The further you are close to start blossoming and become healthier, stronger, and more confident.

# Conclusion

Thanks, another time for getting this precise guide - *Intermittent Fasting for ladies Over 50*.

Women have a bent to be more reactionary, cautionary, and emotional than men. Meaning you're more likely to start out applying the items you've learned in this book and have it make a difference in your life than the typical man if he were to read an identical text.

Before you jump in, I suggest you're taking the time to do more research and take into consideration what you've read then ask yourself why you would like to do this in the first place. Once you've discovered strong reasons to anchor your actions, it'll be easier to maneuver forward once you are faced with difficulties down the road. Because there's no sugar-coating it, you'll meet some rough patches where you'll want to quit. But you're a strong-willed goddess! That's the advantage of learning as an older adult. What most children will face, struggle with, and ultimately contribute the towel, you'll gleefully shine at by drawing on your wealth of experience to beat any hurdle.

Although I even have written this book for all older women, it might be a classic mistake to place you beat one category. You're a singular individual; therefore, approach the suggestions and proposals in this book as a suggestion with flexibility, which will be amended to suit you the simplest. This book was written to offer you a broad perspective on intermittent fasting. It's now your address dip your toe in the water, so to talk, and check out these various methods as a test. Once you find the tactic that resonates with you and suits your specific needs, plan to it. With time, you'll master the tactic and even introduce a couple of changes to make it your customized intermittent fasting plan.

It is the norm for people to undertake out intermittent fasting as an answer to various health problems. However, to urge the foremost out of practice, it's better to approach it as a replacement way. That's to mention, even after achieving your health goal (weight loss, improved cognitive function, balanced hormones, healthier skin), you ought to continue practicing intermittent fasting as a daily a part of your day. Don't throw it all away because you've reached a couple of milestones. Remember that one among the advantages of intermittently fasting is to extend longevity. While you'll not typically follow a rigorous diet plan as you'd in the early stages of fasting, you must maintain these habits to stay reaping its benefits.

When you are in great shape, you'll have things to seem forward to as any healthy woman should, no matter her age. The anticipation of girls is increasing, so why endure a low quality of life for even longer? Never invest the ideas that your body has got to decline with age. Don't just allow the experience to varying; make it change for you!